# Sex Positions for Couples

*Make Your Couple's Sex Life Amazing with The Leading Top Sex Positions and With Techniques and Tips for Awesome Fantasy Time.*

medical or professional advice. The content within this book has been derived from various sources. Please consult a licensed professional before attempting any techniques outlined in this book.

By reading this document, the reader agrees that under no circumstances is the author responsible for any losses, direct or indirect, which are incurred as a result of the use of information contained within this document, including, but not limited to, — errors, omissions, or inaccuracies.

# Table of Contents

# Introduction

First off, I would like to thank you for choosing this book, and I hope that you find it informative and helpful no matter what your needs may be. Congratulations on taking these first steps in improving your sex life. This can be a hard topic for some people, but we are here to strip away all of those awkward feelings about sex. Here, we will celebrate sex as something natural. The goal of the book is to help people improve their sex lives because sex should be something that helps bring couples closer and to improve their overall wellbeing. Sex should not be done only for procreation.

This book will walk you through all of the various aspects of sex and foreplay. The first thing we are going to go over is kama sutra and tantric sex and the benefits of practicing them. These are two common topics that get discussed in the world of sex, but so many people don't actually know what they are or what they even mean. They are not both the same, as you will soon find out, and they will bring something a bit different into your sex life.

Besides that, we are also going to go over how to get your body and mind ready for sex. One of the most common issues people have when it comes to unsatisfactory sex is that they aren't able to get out of their own head enough to really enjoy what is happening. With the right preparation, this doesn't have to be a problem.

Then we will look at some tips that can help out those who may not have all that much experience in sex. Everybody has to begin somewhere, and there is no need to feel ashamed.

After that, the next couple of chapters are going to go over the various ways that can get you and your partner ready for sex. We will go over some tantric massage techniques, preliminary games, dirty talk, and other secrets of a good couples massage. These tend to be things that people like to avoid because they are afraid of messing them up, which makes sense, but you won't have to worry about that anymore after you have read this book.

Next, we will go over the orgasm. This is the main goal that everybody is aiming for when having sex, right? So why shouldn't we discuss it and what it means and how to improve your chances of having multiple orgasms? This will naturally bring us into our next subject, female ejaculation. This has been seen as the lost unicorn in the sex world, but we are going to dispel the myths that you may have heard and explain to you exactly what it is.

Then we will move into specific sex positions for you to try. First, we will go over the best sex positions for him, then the best positions for her, and then the best positions to bring both of your closer.

After that, we will look at some exercises that men can use in order to increase their orgasmic control. This is a common issue that men can run into, and it does not mean that they have anything wrong with them. With these exercises, men can learn how to control their orgasms so that they are able to last long enough to please their partner.

Then we will go over the best sex positions to use when your partner is pregnant. Sex during pregnancy is often seen as impossible or tricky, but there are positions out there that can make sex during pregnancy easy. After that, we will go over the best sex positions for oral. Oral sex is often forgotten about, but it can make things more interesting.

Lastly, we will wrap everything up with talking about things that you can do to improve your sex life. While the goal of the entire book is to improve your sex life, these exercises can be used in addition to everything else that we will talk about.

Making a choice to not be stuck in the same monotonous sex every night is a big decision. Having amazing sex should not be a mystery, and with this book, it no longer will be.

Before we begin, I would like to ask that if you find any part of this book helpful and informative, please rate and leave it a review.

# Chapter 1: The Art of Kama Sutra

For many people, when they hear the words "Kama Sutra," they automatically see some contortionist sex positions. They think it requires positions that use acrobatics, yoga, and maybe even some primeval pornography. This is only partly true.

The *Kama Sutra* actually covers much more than what people in the Western world see. To simply say that it is just a book full of spicy sex positions is providing this ancient, sacred Hindu text a disservice.

Kama Sutra isn't something that magically turns everyday sex into sacred lovemaking. That part is only like 20 percent of what it is about. Real, sacred lovemaking is mainly about a deep connection and spirit, which is the reason why the sex positions of the *Kama Sutra* only take up about 20 percent of the text. The rest of it helps to guide you through the art of love. Kama Sutra also helps you with things like:

- Etiquette

- Family life

- Balancing your masculine and feminine energies in yourself and in the partnership

- The philosophy and nature of love

- Proper grooming

- What triggers and sustains desire

- Self-care

- The practice of different arts like poetry, cooking, and mixing

- Many other non-sexual, pleasure-oriented facets of life

It helps you to live a good life and not simply how to have amazing contortionist sex.

Kama Sutra, which is also written as Kamasutra, is a Sanskrit word made of two words, "kama" and "sutra." Both words have different meanings, but when they are combined, the meaning makes up the premise of what Kamasutra is all about.

"Kama" in Sanskrit translates to "desire," and includes both the aesthetic and sensual desires. However, when it comes to Kamasutra, it places emphasis on sensual desire. In the majority of world religions, a person's sexual desire is viewed as taboo.

However, within Hinduism, "kama" is one of the "four goals of Hindu life." Their four goals of life include, "kama," "artha," meaning success and abundance, "dharma," meaning truth and virtue, and "moksha," meaning release.

In Sanskrit, "sutra" means thread or line, but in the sense of Kama Sutra, it is talking about a thread of verses that create a manual.

## Where Does it Come From?

Kama Sutra comes from the ancient Hindu book called the *Kama Sutra* that was written by the Indian philosopher Vatsyayana Mallanaga between 400 to 200 BCE. What is interesting is that Vatsyayana said that he was a celibate monk. He also said that bringing together all of this sexual wisdom was the contemplation of deity and a form of meditation.

Vatsyayana wasn't the teacher of this wisdom but simply composed the Kama Sutra from a book that was written much earlier, in the seventh century, called Kamashastra, or *Rules of Love*. This other book is a lot larger, but it also looked at the love-customs and partner compatibility of Northern India.

The *Kama Sutra* was written in a difficult and complex form of Sanskrit. Even when it was translated to English, the ideas still come off as a bit abstract to the modern reader. Thanks to Bhagwan Lal Indraji and Sir Richard Francis Burton, we can look at the complex translation from the Kama Sutra. This excerpt is about the different varieties of moaning that take place during lovemaking:

*"The whimper, the groan, the babble, the wail, the sigh, the shriek, the sob, and words with meaning, such as 'mother, 'stop,' 'let go,' or 'enough.' Cries like those of doves, cuckoos, green pigeons, parrots, bees, moorhens, geese, ducks, and quails are important options for use in moaning."*

Not exactly what you would think of when it comes to moaning, is it? Luckily, people have studied it more and more translations have been written that make it easier to understand.

## Sex and Beyond

As stated above, Kama Sutra isn't just about sex. For example, a large part of Kama Sutra is about flirting and courtship. It states that if a man wants to attract a woman, he should hold a party and ask his guests to recite poetry. When the poetry is read, people should leave out certain parts, and then the guests compete to complete the poem. It also suggests that the man and woman should play together, meaning they should do things together like swimming.

Kama Sutra also focuses a lot on dating with the aim of getting married. Finding your ideal partner involves making sure that you possess the same qualities that you would like your partner to have.

When it does come to sex and intimacy, Kama Sutra also includes the nonsexual aspects. There are eight categories of embrace. The first four are expressive of mutual love, and the other four are to increase pleasure during intimacy and foreplay.

1.   Touching Embrace

This helps a man and woman get acquainted, develop the hots for one another, and the man feels passion fire up so that he starts looking for an excuse to get closer with the purpose of brushing his body against her.

2.  Piercing Embrace

The piercing embrace happens when a part of the man touches the woman's private parts, such as her breasts, without a known intention, but as an accident. But because of the touch, the man feels an instant sexual urge to grab her breasts when secluded or in the dark.

3.  Rubbing Embrace

When a couple passes each other in the dark or down a lonely alley, or even in public, they realize their sexual attraction towards one another, so they make a point or rubbing their bodies against one another because of their desire to feel each other up.

4.  Pressing Embrace

The rubbing can move to something else that is guided by intense arousal. This happens when one person pushes the other against a wall and presses their body tightly against the other to bring them closer so that they can feel their partner's intimate parts.

5.  Twining of a Creeper (Jataveshtikaka)

This embrace occurs when a woman clings to her man in the way that a creeper twines around a strong plant that stands tall and steady. She then pulls the man's head towards her so that she can kiss him, while intently staring deep into his eyes.

6.  Climbing a Tree (Vrikshadhirudhaka)

This embrace occurs when a woman places a hand around his shoulder, reaching to touch the back of his other shoulder. One of her feet is placed on his thighs, and the other foot is on his feet, just like she was getting ready to climb a tree. These moves show that she wants a kiss from him.

7. Mixture of Sesame Seed with Rice (Tila Tandulaka)

You know what it is like to be laying down and to be spooned or to spoon your partner? This is what this embrace is like. Whether you choose to lay face to face or front to back, you both need to be laying next to one another and have your legs and arms entwined.

8. Milk and Water Embrace (Kshiraniraka)

The act of sex is imminent; you become vulnerable to your partner. This is the type of embrace that happens with a sexual union when two bodies are pressed against one another as tightly as you can like you are entering into one another. The woman should be sitting on his lap, facing him, so that they can feel each other up in the best way possible, enjoying whatever sensations happen.

Besides embracing one another, Kama Sutra also covers kissing. The Kama Sutra actually has 26 forms of kisses that range from kisses to showing affection and respect, to those that are used during sex and foreplay. The best kiss for sexual partners is one that based on being aware of the emotional state of your partner when you two are not having sex.

Other aspects of intimacy and foreplay include mutual massages, rubbing, biting, pinching, and using the hands and fingers to stimulate each other, as well as many different forms of cunnilingus and fellatio.

Kama Sutra is also inclusive of same-sex relationships, as well as sex "games" like group sex and BDSM.

# Chapter 2: Benefits of Kama Sutra

Everybody understands that changing up sex positions and trying new things is good for their sex life. Even still, people choose to stick with what they are used to for one reason or the other. Let's take a moment to look at the benefits of trying new things in bed, specifically Kama Sutra.

- Different Perspective

When you change up your sex positions, you are also changing your perspective in bed. You get to see new areas of your partner's body and experience different types of stimulation.

This is a very important thing for men because their eyes are the second most important zone to his penis. Women love with their ears, but men love with their eyes. Men have visual sex, which is why they are more likely to watch porn. When they get to see something new that is also exciting, it only makes the sex that much better.

For example, in missionary, you only see each other's faces, but if you move to doggy style, he gets a perfect view of her rear end. The same is true if the woman gets on top. They get a nice view of each other's chest.

- Tone The Organism

In Eastern medicine, there is a notion that all parts of the organs and body are connected, and each part can be influenced by another part. Genitals of men and women have many representative areas of every vital organ within the body. During sex, and in various sexual positions, these parts are stimulated. This means that you can be helping other areas of your body when you are having sex.

- Different Sensations

In all the sexual positions that we will talk about in later chapters, the penis will touch a different area of the vagina and enters at varying depths. This changes how sex feels for him and her. For women, they are all different. They feel different things even if they are stimulated in the exact same spot. For men, they feel pretty much the same thing all the time.

- Help Women Reach an Orgasm

The worst thing for a woman is not reaching orgasm during sex. Every woman is unique in what she needs in order to climax, so trying out new things in bed can help her to get exactly what she wants.

Why would you risk your relationship when all you need to do is change up your positions so that she actually has an orgasm? It is important for men to understand exactly how their partner's body works so that they know what she needs.

- Boost In Confidence

Simply following Kama Sutra can help boost a person's self-confidence. The actual *Kamasutra* book provides tips on how to boost a person's confidence and guides you to help make your personality magnetic.

# Chapter 3: Trying Tantric Sex

Tantric sex is probably one of the best things to try out if you want to achieve the biggest orgasm of your life. If you don't believe me, then continue reading, If you do believe me and want to learn how, then continue reading.

Tantric sex is a Hindu practice that dates back more than 5,000 years ago. The word tantra is Sanskrit means "woven together." Buddhist and Hindu meditation practitioners often use the union of tantra as a way to help weave together the spiritual and physical, which also weaves women to men, and the Divine to humanity. The main purpose of the practice is to become one with God. The way that the Western achieves this is by teaching people to have slow intercourse without reaching orgasm.

Couples who have chosen to try tantric sex say that they reached more pleasure and have experienced a sense of "becoming one with each other" that is very loving and profound. The main goal of this sexual practice is to be enlightened and not trying to win a gold medal for gymnastics of the carnal type. If this comes off as a bit confusing, this of it this way. If having a quickie is the sexual equivalent of take out, tantric sex is the Michelin-starred meal, lovingly and slowly prepared and more delicious thanks to the wait.

## Practice Makes Perfect

You will start things out by facing each other and looking deep within your partner's eyes. Your clothes should remain on while doing this. Remain focused only on the other person's eyes. This is going to help keep the two of you intimate. Some people have said that to keep the tension down during this act is to switch up which eye you are looking at, but some consider this to be cheating the practice. Your eyes are the windows to your soul. The point of this act is that the two of you are gazing into each other's souls.

Check in with your breathing. Yes, you could be breathing wrong during this practice. You should try to get your breathing synchronized with your partners. You both should be breathing in at the same time and then breathing out at the same time. Then you will transition into what is known as breath exchange. You will breathe in as your partner breathes out, and then you will breathe out when they breathe in. This is meant to mimic you breathing into each other. This should be practiced for about ten minutes before moving on.

## For Starters

To transition this into tantric sex, you will do the same thing described above but without any clothes on. You are going to sit in your partner's lap, facing them. Next, you will wrap your legs around their waist and start to practice your breath exchange. Now you will start to caress and kiss each other. After some time, penetration can take place, and the two of you can start very slow intercourse. Make sure that you continue to caress and kiss one another. Your eye contact should be maintained through all of this.

Now things get to get a bit more interesting. Once the two of you get more proficient, you could actually build the ability to have longer orgasms. For men and women alike, this is a different way of having multiple orgasms. This will make you remain at the top of your pleasure without actually having an orgasm. You will get to enjoy all of the same feelings as having an orgasm, but it can help you last for several minutes, or even hours, without ever having a regular orgasm. This is able to create an emotional merging, as well as profound sex. There are some women who have been able to have an orgasm while doing specific exercises.

## Other Ways to Tantra

What we have gone over is only one way to perform tantric sex. The good news is, tantric sex isn't really goal oriented, so there isn't a right or wrong way to do it. The trick of tantra is to take your mind off of the orgasm and focusing on making foreplay more enjoyable and rewarding until you are both ready to reach its natural end. This is often easier said than done, so in order to delay orgasm, tantric experts offer different methods such as massage, breath control, and meditative techniques.

The first thing you can do is to start by turning down the lights and shutting out the world around you. Loosen up your body. Tantra focuses on moving the energy through your body, so you should shake your limbs vigorously to help energize and unblock your body before you get started.

You may also want to stay off of the bed. Sometimes getting onto the bed will trigger your sleep button, which means that you two will choose to have a quick romp instead of a deep connection and loving sex, which is the goal of tantra.

You can try to lay down with your partner on the floor, with some blankets and pillows to make it more comfortable, and slowly start to touch one another. Take your time to leisurely make your way across their body.

Start experimenting with different types of touches, such as gentle strokes, light feathery touches, and firm massages. The aim of this is to heighten each other's senses in a slow and intense way so that you can build each other to a peak but not taking each other all the way. When done the right way, this is able to prolong the sex and your pleasure for hours.

If you start to find that your mind is wandering, refocus yourself on your breaths. Practice the breath exchange that was discussed earlier. This will help to keep your both focused and bring you closer together.

Above all else, don't give up. The first time you try this, don't be surprised if you don't last more than ten minutes or so. Try again. Tantric sex is going to take some time to get the grip of because we have all become used to our western way of sex. This means that we all expect sex to have an obvious beginning, middle, and end.

## Tips and Tricks

Tantra isn't a one-size-fits-all practice. There are different things you can do to improve your practice and to make it more satisfying and unique.

- You don't have to get naked. You can begin things while clothed, and you can remain clothed, or you can choose to remove all of your clothing. The important thing is to do whatever feels comfortable for both of you. This will look very different for everybody.

- Focus on your breathing. Deep breathing is a very important part of tantric sex. When you focus on your breath, it gives you the chance to be present in the moment and to fully immerse yourself in the experience.

- Use all of your senses. Light a few scented candles. Play some sensual, soft music. Slowly touch your partner. Start into one another's eyes. Savor the taste of the kiss. Engage every sense during your tantric practice, and this will help you to feel every ounce of pleasure more fully.

- Go at things slowly. An important part of tantra is to learn how to feel and experience things on a deeper level. The best way to achieve this is to go slowly. You shouldn't rush tantra. Instead, you need to relax your mind and enjoy every second.

- Explore everything area of your partner's body. Stroke you hands slowly over their body. Use your tongue to explore their mouth as you kiss. You can also gently glide your lips up and down their chest. Let them do the same thing to you.

- You can experiment with things as well. For example, kink and BDSM often incorporate tantric ideas. When you are practicing tantra, there is no rule that says you have to stick to traditional practices. You can think outside of the box.

- There is no need to go full tantra. You can add in elements of tantric practices into your bedroom game. This could mean meditation as part of foreplay or focusing more on your deep breathing to help slow things down.

## The Importance of Reconnecting

With our lives constantly being over-scheduled, we don't make sure that we take the time to stop and stay focused on our partners. Couples have come to realize that a normal monogamous relationship isn't working for them anymore. There are some couples who decide to have an open relationship for this reason alone. Performing tantric sex is a way to enhance your sexual pleasures and the relationship in several different ways. First, when you emphasize the breath, it helps to connect both of you on a more intimate and deeper level. This alone is able to help open your heart up to being more forgiving, loving, and closer to your sexual partner.

Second, since tantric sex is performed at such a slow pace, this will give you the chance to see how sensual your mind and body can be. Being able to enjoy sex for an hour or more is equivalent to turning a single taco from a fast-food restaurant into a Mexican feast. Either one is going to take care of your hunger, but that feast is going to provide you with more pleasure, satisfaction, and delight.

Last but certainly not least, you may not enjoy the thoughts of not having an orgasm, but his can help both of you create connectedness and ecstasy beyond the normal orgasm.

# Chapter 4: Getting Ready for Sex

The secret to an invigorating sex life lies within the mind. Do you remember when sex seemed like a seven-course feast? You didn't know what was coming next, every mouthful made you tingle from head to toe, and once you reached the end of it, you felt content and satisfied. Nowadays, it seems like a bowl of cereal; convenient, quick, and fills a gap, but it's not something you would want to have every single day.

In order to get great sex back, you need to put it on the brain. When you make sure that you turn your brain on before you have sex, it will trigger your libido. Let's take a moment to look at some ways to get your mind ready for sex.

## Take It Slow

How come a man can go from watching a slasher film to hopping into bed and instantly feeling horny, but a woman hops into bed and starts to think about everything they have to do the next day? The female brain and the male brain work differently. A woman's brain works by multitasking, but a man's brain typically focuses on one thing at a time.

Studies have found that a woman needs a transition time of 10 to 30 minutes between activities. That means that if you want to have sex before going to sleep at night, turn off the television and take some time before jumping into bed. During this time, you could have a warm aromatherapy bath or a massage to help put one another in the mood. The best scents for arousal are sandalwood, bergamot, chamomile, or lemon.

## Just Say Yes

For some, having sex can be like having to go to the gym. Their body and mind start to rebel against is, but once they do it, they feel great. Standard wisdom has said, for a woman, the sexual cycle goes from desire to arousal, to orgasm. There has been new research that has found that women who are in long-term relationships will experience desire after they become aroused. That means, sometimes, you simply have to be receptive to your partner's touch instead of giving in to the voice that's telling you to go to sleep.

When you give into that touch, your brain will start to focus on pleasures that follow and will then increase the blood flow to the right areas. Even if all you have is a quickie and you don't orgasm, the biochemicals released during sex are still released, which will help you to want to have more sex, more often.

There are ways for women to help get themselves aroused instead of waiting on their partners to initiate. You can start by tensing your pelvic floor muscles. All of these muscles support your pelvic floor, as well as your genitals, and helps to stimulate the arousal process.

## Morning Person

While most people think about having sex right before bed, mornings are actually the best time for sex. This is the time of day when your body has produced more sex hormones, such as testosterone. If setting aside time in the morning to have sex is out of the question, you should still use those early-morning hormones to help get your mind ready for a night of passion. Simply thinking about sex during the day can often be enough to make you want it.

That means, instead of just giving your partner a peck goodbye, take some time to look deep into their eyes and then give them a long lingering kiss. Wrap things up by whispering, "Our room, 10 pm." This will not just leave your partner anticipating the night to come, but it will also turn you on.

Getting the mind ready is only part of getting ready for sex. You also want to make sure that your body is ready as well.

## Fantasy

You can also use your mind to help trigger your desire for your partner. There is a simple exercise you can do for this. You and your partner sit across from one another, hold hands, and then stare into one another's eyes. Don't say a word, but both of you should start to think about the last time that you had sex and really enjoyed it. This helps to create a connection between the mind and body. It works a lot like how you shiver when you recall a scary experience. When focusing on all the little sexy details, it will ignite your body and turn you on. You will also get to see the arousal on your partner's face.

## Get Some Sleep

There is nothing worse than falling asleep before sex. One of the main reasons why new parents lose their sex lives is that they are too tired. Sex just doesn't sound good when you haven't had enough sleep. If you have noticed that you are too tired to get intimate, you need to make sure that you make sleep a priority. Make sure that you are getting the recommended seven to nine hours each night. To improve your sleep, you should make sure all devices are turned off.

## Ask Questions

One of the most common reasons why you may be turning your partner down is out of boredom. This boredom doesn't have to do with just positions. You also have to rediscover what you both want. You should always ask questions, like: "Do you like it when I do this?" This will help you to feel more comfortable and confident when it comes to asking for what you want. You should also feel comfortable looking outside of your own bedroom for new inspiration.

## Talk To Your Doctor

This tends to apply more for women, but men, feel free to talk to your doctor if you haven't been experiencing any sexual desire. For women, you should speak with your gynecologist if you have noticed that you have been having a hard time getting turned on for your partner. There are medical reasons that could cause this. Depression, menopause, hormonal imbalance, and some medications can impact your libido. Fortunately, topical and oral medications, lubricants, and hormone therapy can help get your mojo back. You should never feel embarrassed to talk to your doctor about this, that have heard everything.

## Understand Her Cycle

Women are influenced by their cycle. They will find sex more enjoyable at different times of their cycle. From day one to 14, women produce more testosterone, which means it is easier to get turned on and reach climax. Women also experience a surge in libido during days 24 to 28 because of the nerve endings that are stimulated by the thickening of the uterine lining.

## Food

We know a healthy diet is important for a long and healthy life, but the foods you eat can also affect your libido. Foods like honey, peanut butter, and bananas contain vitamin B, which naturally boosts your libido. Celery contains androsterone, which can help aid in female attraction. There are a lot of other foods out there that act as natural aphrodisiacs as well.

## Kick Those Bad Habits

There are already plenty of reasons to stop smoking, but I've got one more for you. Smoking can actually hurt your sex life. Cigarettes narrow the blood vessels, and this makes it harder for the blood to flow to the genital region, which is very important for both men and women when it comes to sexual stimulation. You should also make sure that you don't drink too much. Too much alcohol will act as a depressant and decrease your libido.

If you make sure that you follow at least some of these tips before you have sex, your mind and body will be ready, and one won't let the other down.

## Role Playing

Have you ever felt like you would want to be somebody different behind closed doors? Have you ever felt the need to change up the power dynamics in your relationship? Have you found yourself fantasizing about being a robber, schoolteacher, or police officer? Does it make you feel like you're gross or weird to feel that way?

It shouldn't. Roleplay within a relationship is actually very healthy. In spite of what you might have been told growing up or what might have been said on early morning bad cable shows, sex isn't something that is dirty, and role-play isn't a sinister act that only deviants and sinners indulge in.

Role-play is a healthy practice for couples, married, or otherwise, that can help you to improve and strengthen your connection with your partner. The desire to pretend to be somebody else doesn't have anything to do with dissatisfaction with your partner or sex life. It has to do with safety and trust.

Role-playing is simply the act of acting out your or your partner's fantasies, and this act of playing out fantasies often happens when you feel secure and safe in your relationship. Role-playing is a great indicator of feeling physically and emotionally safe with your partner.

Role-play has the ability to be a healing experience and can help to strengthen the relationship of the individual. It is a great way to express your desires or yourself. While movies and porn may make you think that women and men already have their fantasy roles laid out, that isn't necessarily the case in reality.

For example, if you are the woman in a heterosexual couple and your boyfriend is a high-powered financial analyst, and he wants you to spank him and treat him as a "bad boy," he could be hinting that he doesn't always need to be in control. The two different roles, the submissive and the dominant character in this type of sexual exploration, can change the bonds between people. It can enliven, deepen, and strengthen the relationships, whether you switch between a submissive and dominant role or remain static.

The fantasies you have are a lot more common than you believe. There are three common fantasies:

1.   Public or spontaneous sex

2. Bisexual fantasies

3. Dominant and submissive

Chances are, you have had one of these fantasies before.

For the dom and sub fantasies, it gives you the chance to have an unequal power distribution in a controlled and safe situation. It gives you the chance to release your inhibitions and to be taken over by pleasure, and either have a gain or loss of control.

Humans have a subcortical circuit for submission and dominance. The majority of us will display these two sides several times throughout the day. A partner who would like to be dominant might have, or currently, feels weak and helpless during certain points of their life and benefits from getting to feel as if they are in control in a certain area.

With a bisexual fantasy, simply wanting to role play in a bisexual role, doesn't mean that you actually have homosexual tendencies. This, in no way, means that everybody is bisexual, but a lot of people have experienced sexual interest towards a person of the same gender.

With a spontaneous fantasy, it is one of the "just can't wait to have you" type of things. This is something that we have all heard about and thought about, if not, we've given it a try. The thought of having sex in a public setting can be quite invigorating because of the danger behind it.

There is no need to be afraid of the idea of foreplay. It does not mean that you feel unhappy in your relationship, and it doesn't mean that you think your current sex life is boring. Simply wanting to be another person during sex doesn't mean you are going to hurt your relationship and the life that you both have outside of the bedroom.

The key to having a healthy and successful role-play is trust. Without trust, boundaries may end up being crossed, and your lines can be destroyed. It is all about having mutual respect and a good understanding that this is simply an exploration of fantasies, and the most important element of it all is consent.

Through this act of self-expression, there is an opportunity for validation and acceptance from your partner, which can lead to an intimate and emotional connection. The lowered inhibitions and sexual confidence that is needed when you role play can only be reached through safety and trust in your relationship.

If you are able to engage in role-playing with confidence, you aren't being some sexual pariah. Instead, you are proving that you have faith in your lover and partnership with them. If you can comfortably open yourself up to that level of vulnerability, you are reaffirming your connection.

Roleplay equals communication. When you are in tune with your sexual self, you are traveling an enlightened path. You want to feel relaxed enough in your relationship to feel like you can ask your partner for whatever it is that you want without feeling shameful.

In order to have good communication, you have to be in tune with yourself. Having a good understanding of what you desire and being aware of the level of openness and comfort you have to act out that desire is going to help you talk to your partner. If you have a solid relationship, then this communication should be fluid. So what should you do if you think role playing is for you? Here is where you need to start.

1.   Think About What Your Fantasies Are

First, you each need to figure out what you want. In your head, what turns you on? Is it a teacher you had in college? Maybe you have always wanted a massage therapist to take things a step further. You may have even fantasized about being your favorite book character. Your only limit is your imagination. Think about any type of scenario that turns you on, even if it is something as simple as a first date with a person you have lusted over. Your dirty thoughts are the best inspiration for role-playing games.

2.   Talk About It

There are some fantasies that can happen spur of the moment, like pretending to meet them for the first time. Others are going to need some prep work. If it is something really kinky that involves whips, leather, or some type of costume, you are going to have to give your other half a heads-up.

You can start things off by saying, "I can't stop fantasizing about..." Then you can gauge their interest in it. If you notice they perk up a little or get into it, then you can take things to the next level.

3.  Be Kinky or Not

There are some fantasies that are all about power, such as officer and criminal, or student and teacher. One of you is going to have to have power over the other in some way. This is a great way to explore a power exchange dynamic in a playful way. But not every scenario is going to have the power play. Pretending to pick them up in a bar, or acting as if you are on a blind date gives you the chance to be somebody that you don't think you are, such as overtly sexual, aggressive, or bold.

4.  Start Slow

For some, role playing is going to feel silly. You may feel uncomfortable or awkward "playing pretend," even if it is something that turns you on. This is why it is best to begin slowly and with something small. You may try sexting about your fantasy at first. This gives you the chance to be imaginative without having to look at the other person or speaking. For some, this is all they want or need. For others, after they get comfortable with typing things, it is going to be easy to say their "lines" as the scene plays out.

5.  Dress Up or Not

Imagination is extremely powerful, so costumes aren't always needed. If you aren't interested in buying costumes and the like, then skip it. But if the act of dressing up helps you get into your role, then go for it. If you aren't sure if you need the costume or not, try it with the costume and without to see which way you prefer.

There are a lot of places to buy costumes online. There are adult stores that you can buy things from, and you can also try Halloween stores, especially when they have their sales after Halloween has passed. You may even find some things in your closet that will work.

6.  What Do I Say?

The first few things that you say as your character may seem silly or awkward, and that is okay. This is something new, and nobody expects you to be perfect when you first start out. It is okay to fumble and laugh. If the fantasy has a strong connection for you and your partner, then the words will come and you can follow each other's lead.

You might know how you would like things to end. If you do, you need to tell your partner. But you might also want to be surprised; in which case you should imagine what your character would say and go with it. There isn't a critic in your house that is going to tell you what you should and should not do. If the role play ends with both of you naked, sweaty, and satisfied, then you have done well.

# Chapter 5: Beginner Sex Tips

If you took the time to compare your sex life to today's dating scene, you might think your sex life is blander than mashed potatoes. That said, you should never get "wild" just because that is what everybody on TV is doing. Research has found that spontaneity and openness are able to lead to a longer-lasting relationship. Don't let other people mess with your mind.

After you have gotten used to talking candidly about sex with your significant other about what you want to try out and what you don't, it will become a lot easier to do in the future. A lot of people prefer to have a partner who feels empowered. This is going to help you to build respect and improve communication between the two of you. So, for those of you who are still new to improving your sex life, or haven't really gotten started with your sex life, let's go over some tips on how you can make some changes.

- Casually Mention It

Every sex expert out there will tell you that if you are having problems talking with your significant other about your sex life, you can let a song, erotic book, or movie provide you with inspiration. The conversation can easily be started with, "I saw this movie," or "I read an article about..." After that, you can let the conversation naturally continue.

- Don't Be Afraid to Be The Initiator

If your partner is normally the one that initiates sex, change things up a bit by showing them how much they excite you and flip the switch so that you can get things started. Everybody loves to feel as if their partner can't resist them.

- Practice Some Non-Sexual Touch

While this may have more to do with putting in some work when you aren't having sex, it can end up leading to an overall better sex life. You shouldn't reserve touching for solely when you are naked. Find a way to add in some hand holding, back rubs, hair stroking, and any other non-sexual touching that will encourage you and your partner to show affection for each other. You will learn more about each others' bodies in a way that is a lot deeper than simply have sex.

- Toys

If you would like to experiment with some toys, begin with simple ones. The easiest one to try is a vibrating ring. They fit over the penis and can be used with a condom. Most guys like these because, well, they vibrate of course. They also provide stimulation for the clitoris, so it really won't matter which position you are in, everybody wins. It isn't just pleasurable for one or the other.

Even if there isn't a penis around, vibrating rings can be used as a massager. You don't have to use them on the genitals.

- No Toys, No Problem

Even though it is exciting when you introduce new things into the relationship, you don't have to have toys to increase the heat.

It isn't always about bringing things into the bedroom. It could be about changing up the location. It might be an erotic book or porn. It might be creating a playlist of songs that turn you on. After two songs, anything might happen.

The most important thing is you don't need to make it complicated. Try to find just a few phrases that you think you can pull off and try them out first. If talking seems too hard, just begin by getting more verbal when you are having sex. Moans and groans can help you get used to being more vocal during sex. This will also help your partner know they are going things that you like.

- Lubes

The easiest thing to add to your sex life is lubricants. Water-based lubes are easier to clean up since the main component is water. These are normally cheaper. There is one drawback to this type of lube. They normally dry up faster than the silicone-based ones. The silicone-based ones last longer and are thicker. If you are having sex underwater, you are going to need a lube that won't wash off. If you are trying anal sex, where lube is very important, silicone-based lubes are your best option.

- Remember to Communicate

This one should be a no brainer, but anytime you begin pushing the boundaries in the bedroom, you have to make sure your partner is consenting to the new things.

If you are into any type of verbalizing or fantasy play that is going to involve your partner saying stop, they need to be able to do that. Everyone needs a safe word. Although you aren't into discipline or bondage, you might need some way to tell your partner it's time to stop.

If your significant other wants to do something you aren't into, say something like: "I appreciate you telling me about your fantasy, and I would like to explore it by talking about it. Right now, it isn't anything that I would be willing to actually try." When you let your partner know that you aren't comfortable with it, you are letting them know that there isn't anything wrong with their fantasy. They don't need to feel ashamed or guilty about asking about it.

Basically, sex is all about what is and isn't pleasurable and comfortable for your partner and yourself. There isn't any way to be an advanced sexual partner. When you have sex with your partner, if it is fulfilling and fun, then it is perfectly fine. Never do anything new just to keep away from a breakup.

Anything you explore needs to be done to enhance your relationship. You need to build on everything you have already created.

# Chapter 6: A Massage to Get Ready

Massages are a great way to get rid of any tension you may have, spread healing energies, improve your blood circulation, and when we are talking about tantra, they can help to sexually arouse your partner. Massages are the best way to help sexual partners show one another extra intimacy.

By nature, humans crave touch, and massages are a natural and an easy way to get that much-needed human touch. So how can you achieve this? First, there is no need to head out and get some special certification or training to help you perform your tantric massages. The only thing you really need is to have a yearning and intention to genuinely satisfy your partner through the intricate capacities of your hands.

## What Does Tantric Massage Mean?

Before we head into the actual massage techniques, we should go over what a tantric massage is, how it differs from other types of massages and the biggest benefits of it. The tantric massage that we will go over was first created from many different sources, which are mainly a mixture of tantric philosophy and influences from the most important Western thinkers.

The main parts of tantric massage include:

- Experiencing a spiritual awakening is the true and ultimate goal of the practice of tantra and tantric massage.

- You should never wear clothes during the massage, so private parts will, the majority of the time, be exposed.

- It helps to heighten or boost orgasmic or sexual experiences.

- It helps to get rid of blockages in various areas of your spirit, mind, body, and consciousness.

- Tantric massage is focused on using and the potential of your sexual energy so that it will benefit you and won't limit you.

## Benefits of Tantric Massage

Just like with any type of massage, a tantric massage comes with many different benefits, as well as some added benefits that make the tantric massage all the more special. The main benefits of having a massage are:

- Increased wellbeing

- Relieves stress, anxiety, and pain

- Improves the mood

- Improves immunity and health

When it comes to tantric massages, you all get these benefits:

- Higher spiritual awareness

- More intense sexual experiences

- Improves sex drive and libido

With all of that out of the way, let's take a look at some techniques and tips to help you get started with your tantric massages.

## Getting Things Setup

For those who have never gotten to have a tantric massage, the thought of a tantric massage is often intriguing, if not intimidating. There are some people who think it is taboo, which is an unfortunate byproduct of our society.

Then you have those who have received a tantric massage, and they see it as a unique, irreplaceable, and exciting practice that can do a lot for a person and their significant other's wellbeing. Since most people don't understand what it is and how it works, they don't even view it as an option for them.

In order to have a good tantric massage session, you are going to want you and your partner to take turns massaging each other. This type of massage is going to require the receiver to be completely open and receptive and to be fully willing to surrender themselves to the experience completely.

To help get things underway, the following are some ways to get things prepared before you get started with the massage.

- Get The Space Ready

You are going to want to get the room where the massage will take place ready. This can be any private space you have in your home, like the bedroom or living room. Make sure that you have plenty of comfortable bedding and soft pillows at your disposal. You can also set the mood by adding some candles, and you can use scented candles to help increase the mood. Make sure that you place your candles in safe areas, away from anything flammable, because the last thing you will want to do is set something on fire in the middle of a massage. Turn the lights off or dim them slightly.

You should also make sure you have something drink nearby, like water or wine. You can also have some light snacks close by to help keep your energy up. You can even feed each other. An oil diffuser can be used to give your room a fresh and soothing scent.

- Get Yourself Fully Prepared

Before you get the massage started, make sure that your mind and heart are open. If you have something that is causing you any sort of discomfort, it is a good idea to try to avoid bringing that up right now, but it might be a good idea to take some time to work through your problems in order to relax further. The main discomfort that people will experience is due to self-consciousness and insecurity about different areas of their body. While you massage one another, it is extremely important to keep your attitude playful and show them you are interested in discovering new interactions.

You may also want to take a shower or a bath before you start the massage. It is a good idea to do this together, but make sure that you stay away from any sexual interactions during your shower. Once that is done, stand face to face and stretch to get rid of tension.

You need to also be wearing comfortable clothing. Make sure that whatever you have on is loose enough that you can take it off easily. However, doing all of this fully nude is a very good idea. Since tantra is about the slow accumulation of sexual energy, it is okay to begin things with your clothes on.

- Start by Slowly Building Sexual Energy

After you have taken your shower and you have stretched, sit down so that you are face to face and in a comfortable position. This could mean that you are cross-legged, or you could have your legs draped over one another in order to help the energy from your erogenous zones to be closer.

Simply sit like this and start into each other's eyes for at least five minutes. As we talked about in the tantric sex chapter, the eyes are the most important part. This will likely feel uncomfortable when you first do this but carry on and stare at each other as long as you can. As you begin to feel all of your tension fall away, you have created a real connection. This is what the goal is of this exercise. This is the connection that you have to have so that you can revel in the tantric massage and sex. Do your best to make sure that you don't lose eye contact during this.

## Begin the Massage

After you are fully ready, whoever wants to receive the massage first can lay down on the surface that you prepared. There are a couple of simple massage methods that you can use, and all of them are beginner-friendly so that you can use them right away. You will want to have some massage oils to make these massages more enjoyable.

- Start on The Back

Add about two tablespoons of massage oils in your hands. Smear the oil across your hands and then rub them together so that you can get the oil and your palms warmed. This will feel better for your partner. Once you have warmed your hands, place them on their low back and let your hands move up their back, over the neck and shoulders, and then back down the back over the butt.

- The Hand Slide

Now that there is a good layer of oil over your partner's back, you can begin to slide your fingers down the spine and then massage all the way down their low back and over their buttocks. Then make your way back up to their neck, over the should, and down their arms and across their fingertips. Do this around five times. As you are massaging them, communicate with them and ask for some feedback on how all of this feels or what they like about it. If your partner doesn't like to talk a lot, you don't have to push them to talk. You need to remember that this is supposed to give them a sense of relaxation and wellbeing.

- Pull-Ups

To change up the motions, try moving one hand after the other as you move up the sides of your lover's body. Start by placing your hands at their hips with your fingertips pointed towards their spine and then pull your hand up to their spine. Once you do both sides, move your hands to their waist, and make the same motion to bring your hand to their spine. Then move your hands up to the side of their breast and pull your hands up to their spine. Lastly, start at their armpits and pull your hands up to their spine. You want to do both sides with each of these.

- Kneading

This is a crazy easy motion, especially for those who have every baked bread. Even if you haven't made bread, it is still a straight forward movement. All you need to do is squeeze their back and buttocks between your fingers and thumbs in a sinuous motion. Then you will allow your hands to glide to another area of their back and then repeat this action over and over until your kneaded all the way up their back. Then you can move your way back down. When you are working in fleshier areas, such as the butt, you can add a little more pressure, so you shouldn't about squeezing it a bit more and spreading their cheeks as your knead.

- Feather Stroke

Before you move down to their thighs, lightly stroke their shoulders, arms, neck, back, and butt with only your fingertips using an extremely light stroke. You should do this for around five minutes. If you have long fingernails, feel free to lightly scratch their skin. You should do this in circular motions and from side to side. The goal is to have this light and prickly touch to create sensual eagerness for your lover because they don't know what area you are going to touch next.

- Foot Caress

You might need to use a bit more oil for this. Rub your oily hands together and then rub the oil down and across their thighs and calves slowly. Knead the back of their legs as well. Do one leg at a time. The feet, whether you realize it or not, is an erogenous zone, so make sure you give them some considerable attention. Add some extra oil to each foot, rubbing it over the ankles, heels, and between the toes. Using the palms of your hands, slide them along the bottom of your partner's foot a few times. Gently rotate their toes clockwise and counter-clockwise. Then move your forefinger between each toe. Gently pull the toes away from the body.

- Flip Them Over

Your partner is probably feeling pleasured after everything you just did to their back, so now you can bring the attention to their front. Have them flip over as you apply more oil to your hands. Smear the oil over their belly and slowly start to slide up their stomach, over their nipples, and then back down to their belly. Continue to do this a few more times. As you do this, it spreads energy into their bodies. If your partner is a female, make sure that you a gentle with her breasts. Men can handle firmer strokes across their chest. You can also knead a man's chest if you want.

Once you have finished massaging your partner, it's your turn to get massaged. Allow the massages to progress naturally and let what happens next, happens. People who are more experienced in tantra and tantric massages will also use yoga poses during their massages. You don't have to use yoga poses in order to have a successful tantric massage.

# Chapter 7: Getting Things Started

The most wonderful thing about playing sex games is that they are all foreplay. Does anybody actually have to justify making sex more intimate, longer-lasting, creative, and playful?

What is foreplay? Foreplay is any type of sexual activity before you have intercourse. With that said, intercourse doesn't even have to be on the menu or the grand finale. Foreplay is hot enough when it is done right. Most women call it "the whole point of having sex." It doesn't matter if it involves a quick text, back rubs, dirty talk, dry humping, spanking, fingering, oral sex, neck kisses, touching each other while spooning, or making out, foreplay is all the sensual things you do before the "huge event," whatever this might mean for you.

Why is foreplay important? There are many reasons why foreplay is so important. It is important for women to feel turned on and excited enough to enjoy sex. Jumping into sex without leading up to it can feel painful, uncomfortable, and boring. Even if you only have time for a quickie, it needs to have some type of lead in so it can be fun for everyone.

You don't go jogging without warming up first, do you? That is all well and good, but it won't get you heated up for sex. All the talking, kissing, touching, and rubbing before sex is just as important as the sex itself. It can help get the blood going to all the right places, boosts the libido, gets you in the mood, and relaxes you. If it is done right, you are going to get your partner primed for an exquisite orgasm.

This definition makes it seem like penetrative intercourse is the only definition of sex. It is best to call it "arousal activities." There are LGBTQ couples who don't actually penetrate each other, and they consider things such as oral sex to be the main event. So, when you call oral sex foreplay, it can be a noninclusive way to look at sex. When you look at foreplay as an appetizer and not the main meal can make it sound like it isn't as important as the man's orgasm.

You should think about foreplay as any activity that can build up arousal, whatever it might be. Sex doesn't need to be a linear experience that begins with a kiss and ends with sex.

As long as all parties involved consent, there isn't a right or wrong way to do foreplay. If oral sex is the main event, then the rubbing and touching that leads to it will give you the arousal you need. Any activity that can get a person "aroused enough to have fun with the other stuff" is considered foreplay.

Here are some classic foreplay activities:

- Spank your partner

- Tell her you enjoy reading her poetry

- Play with your partner's testicles

- Tell him that you love when he plays his guitar (or whatever instrument he might play)

- Nibbling your partner's earlobes

- Fingering your partner's anus

- Biting and kissing your partner's neck

- Fingering her vagina

- Sucking and licking nipples

- Caressing your partner's body all over

- French kissing

- Kissing and licking your partner's anus

- Squeezing and caressing your partner's breasts

- Stroking her penis

- Stroking his penis

You can focus on certain body parts like the back of your partner's neck or their pubic bone. The main part is taking the pressure off of yourself and making your partner have an orgasm. If it feels good for everyone involved, then you are on the right track.

Foreplay can trigger physical and physiological responses that make sex possible and enjoyable.

## Physical Responses

Foreplay can actually get the juices flowing because it increases your sexual arousal. Don't confuse this with sexual desire, but it can do that, too.

Sexual arousal can cause many responses from your body; these include:

- Increases blood pressure, pulse, and heart rate

- Lubricates the vagina. This makes intercourse enjoyable and prevents pain.

- Dilates the blood vessels in the genitals.

- Makes the nipples hard and causes the breasts to swell.

- Blood will flow to the genitals, which in turn cause the penis, clitoris, and labia to swell.

## Physiological Responses

Foreplay does feel good, but it goes a lot deeper than that. When you engage in foreplay, it can help build emotional intimacy that makes you and your significant other feel connected both in and outside the bedroom.

If you aren't in a relationship, no need to worry; foreplay can lower your inhibitions, and this makes sex even hotter between virtual strangers and couples.

If stress halts your libido, foreplay just might take care of this problem. When you kiss, it releases serotonin, dopamine, and oxytocin. This cocktail can lower your cortisol levels while increasing your feelings of euphoria, bonding, and affection.

## Foreplay Means Something Different for Everyone

When talking about sex, foreplay has been defined as an erotic stimulation that precedes sex. If you take sex completely out of the equation, then foreplay becomes defined as a behavior or action that precedes these events

Whatever this event is might not look the same to someone else as it does to you, and this is fine.

You don't even have to put intercourse on the menu if you don't want to. Foreplay is its own thing, and it could be all you need to have an orgasm. If fact, research shows that women can't reach an orgasm just by having sex.

As long as all parties are consenting, foreplay could be anything that you want it to be. You can begin before things get heated up. You need to begin somewhere, but why does it have to be during sex. You don't even have to be in the same room to start.

You can use foreplay to prolong your playtime. If you know that you will be getting together in a couple of days or later today, you can use foreplay to start the party and keep going. Below you will find some foreplay tips. You can find one that you really like and try it out on your partner or get adventurous and try them all. The time you spend on your partner's body

54

before penetration increases their pleasure along with yours when the main course happens.

You don't even have to be in a relationship to play sex games that are intended to be used as couples. Anybody who doesn't mind getting closer would be a great candidate for sex games.

When you find yourself needing to break the ice or get closer, take a look at these ideas for sex games.

- Who's More Powerful

This could be a thumb war, wrestling match, pillow fight, or tickle war. The main thing is you have to do it completely naked. The point of this game is competing, getting each other all worked up, and struggling against your significant other. Whatever the case, the person who surrenders first, has to do a sex act on the other. You need to make sure you agree to the act before you begin. Your partner might not like losing, and you might pick something that they don't like doing.

- Leave notes

You don't have to be creative to get your partner going. You can just leave them a note. Put it on their pillow or hide it in their bag. This shows that you can't wait to be with them later.

- Hide and Seek

This is definitely an R-rated version of the children's game. When you know that your significant other is coming home for the day, take your clothes off and leave a trail for them to follow. Make sure the clothes lead to where you are. Once they open the door and see the clothes, give them time to find you. The best part is they get to decide what happens next. You can then switch roles if you would like to.

- Sexting

Foreplay doesn't have to begin in the bedroom. It can begin when you wake up. This is so easy, and you can do it anytime and anywhere. A text telling them what you want to do to them or how hot you get just thinking about them. You can also tell them certain things they can do to get you all hot and bothered. This shows then that you are thinking about them and everyone loves that. Send them a text that says: "Can't wait to get naked with your later" can get your significant other excited before you ever get into the bedroom. If you are careful, you can even send them a nude picture of you to show them what they can expect later.

- Pick Your Tool

Let your partner try to bring you to orgasm by using a toy or object of your choice. This makes for some great foreplay whether you orgasm or not.

- Meeting For Drinks or Dinner

When you meet your partner for drinks or dinner, make out quickly in the parking lot before you go inside. Once you are inside, play footsies under the table, meet in the restroom for another make-out session. You could "accidentally" drop your fork to take a peek at what they might be wearing under their clothes. These are just a few ways to turn drinks and dinner into foreplay.

- Santa's Bag

If you have any sex toys, put them in a bag. Just make sure they are clean. Ask your significant other to reach into the bag without looking and get one. Whatever toy they pick out is the one that gets used for the night. This keeps either partner from feeling self-conscious about adding a toy to sex.

- Kiss Them Like You Mean It

Don't greet them with a chaste kiss on the cheek. Lock eyes with them, press your body against theirs, and kiss them deep and long.

Use your hands and tongue, and be sure to moan enough to make them excited about what is about to happen. Don't forget to end the night with another fabulous kiss.

- Buy an Adult Board Game

There are more of these on the market than you might think. Some will use cards. Others take a pair of dice. Some games are more traditional. There are some games out there that incorporate all three.

You could get a Jenga set if you don't have on already. Take each block and write down a command like "kiss my neck" and keep going from there. When you play with your partner, whoever extracts a block successfully from the tower, their partner has to perform the command. You can also come up with a punishment from when the tower gets knocked down. You can get naughty and creative on the punishment.

- Tell Them It Is Game Time

You don't have to be coy when all you want to do is get them naked and make wild passionate love to them. Tell them as graphically as you can that all you want to do is get them hot and wet or hard and keep them there all night long.

- Red Light, Green Light

This is not the game you remember from your childhood. You are going to lay down on your bed either naked or in something that makes you feel like a goddess. Have your partner stand at the door to the bedroom. You get to see how well they know you by asking them questions about you. The questions can be anything from personal to sexy. You could ask things like: "Where is my dream vacation?" or "What is my favorite sex position?"

When they get the answer right, they can take a step toward you. If they get the answer wrong, they have to take a step backward. Your significant other is going to learn more about you while going crazy with your teasing. When your partner finally gets to you, let the fun begin.

- Light Candles

There isn't anything like candles to set the mood for all the sexy things you want to do. Tea lights don't cost a lot of money, so stock up and light them when you want to get busy. Plus, candlelight makes your skin look great.

- Timed Penetration

Find some sort of timer. You could use your cell phone, hourglass, or stopwatch. Now choose a time. It could be 30 minutes, ten minutes, or an hour. Now get busy with your partner any way you want. The kicker is there can't be any type of penetration before the time runs out. Once the timer goes off, have all the fun you can handle.

- Turn Music On

Everyone has a song or two that touches them in their special place. You need to find out what your significant other's is and add your to it to create a playlist that will get them all hot and bothered.

Here are a few of my personal favorites:

   o The Weekend – Earned It

   o Nine Inch Nails – Animal

   o Barry White – Let's Get It On

- o  Donna Summer – Love to Love You

- Play Truth or Dare

This one is old, but it's still good. You might need to focus on the dares more than the truth. It all depends on your mood. If you think that they might be hiding something, by all means, stick to the truth but be careful, it might blow up in your face and not in a good way. You could dare your partner to try to kiss you without using their hands. Try to pleasure you by only using the tip of your tongue; this is the best time to uncover all your fantasies.

- Dance

There isn't anything hotter than two bodies being pressed against each other. Feeling your partner's hot breath on your cheek while you sway to the rhythm of your sexy playlist can up the heat factor in the room.

- Mirror

You and your partner need to sit down while facing each other. Start by touching, licking, kissing, or lightly touching your partner. Now they have to repeat what you did to them to you as close as possible to what you did to them. This can get very hot. It's a great way to communicate with them about what you like without actually having to talk to them. Then you get to switch roles. This also helps you pay attention to each other better.

- Sexy Underwear

These aren't just for women. If you can find the right one that fits perfectly, you can really turn your partner on. Low rise briefs are always a good choice.

- Make Out Time

You can go old school and make out. Press your partner up against a wall, get them in the back seat of the car, or just fool around on the couch.

- Striptease

I'm not talking about swinging around a pole. You don't even need to have moves. Just dim the lights, put on your playlist, and slowly take your clothes off. Make sure your expression doesn't show any signs of fear or uneasiness. You can totally fake confidence.

- Make An Erotic Picnic

Place a picnic on your bed that is full of sexy goodies that are meant to be shared. Juicy cherries and strawberries along with some chocolate sauce and whipped cream to dip them into can make for a fun night. You can feed each other and then lick each other clean. Chocolate is a natural aphrodisiac, too.

- Slowly Remove Their Clothes

Since foreplay isn't a sprint, it is a marathon. You aren't in a hurry to get finished. Rather than stripping all your clothes off and getting down and dirty, begin by taking off your partner's shirt. Wait a few minutes and then take their pants off, then remove her bra, etc. until they are completely naked. As you remove an article of clothing, focus on the skin that was revealed. After you take their pants off, you can massage their legs. When the shirt is gone, lick and kiss their chest.

- Massage

Human touch is powerful, and a massage can work wonders on the mind and body. Light those candles and get out your massage oils. There are some massage candles that can be used as both.

Begin at their feet and move up their body. Make sure to hit all their sensual points and linger in those special places when you feel like it.

You can begin by massaging your partner's legs from their upper thighs to their ankles. Now, focus on their feet, kneading their heels and all the parts of their feet. Now, work on their toes. Pull on each of them separately. You get bonus points if you suck them.

A bit of warning here, my partner hates having their feet touched, so you might want to ask their permission before you touch their feet.

- Quality not Quantity

If you can improve the quality of foreplay, she won't ever bug you again about quantity. If you just act like you are going through the motions to have sex with your partner, they will notice, and it is going to take longer to get them excited.

Basically, do what you would like to do and enjoy it; if you like her calves, stroke them. If you love how her butt looks in those jeans, kiss it, or give it a smack. When a man loves what he is doing, it will show, and this will turn her on even more.

- Erogenous Zones

A body is full of hot spots that beg to be touched. Nibble, lick, and kiss your way through all their zones.

- Find Out What Turns Them On

If you have any doubts, just ask them what they want. Most women really appreciate it when their partner makes sure that they are satisfied. If they see that you are trying very hard to please them, they will return the favor.

- Skin to Skin

You might remember dry humping from your teen years. Well, it isn't just for teens. The anticipation of two bodies rubbing together in different states of undress is the hottest thing ever.

- Toys

There is a lot more to sex toys than just a dildo shaped like a penis. Vibrators of various sizes and shapes can be used outside the body on any of the erogenous zones.

You can also find nipple and finger vibrators that can take foreplay to a whole new level.

- Sensory Play

All that dry humping and kissing is probably going to get the job done, but you can take it even farther with some props. Put a blindfold on your partner and then tease them with various temperatures and textures by using your tongue, ice cubes, feathers, etc.

- Tell Them What You Want

Talking about what you want during sex isn't just for foreplay. This makes sure you get what you need and want. Tell them what you want them to do to you and what turns you on.

- Soapy Shower

How wet hands and skin sliding across one another's bodies while you are lathering each other up with soap can take showering to a new level. You might not even want to get out of the shower, ever.

It's amazing at all the things you can find at home, or you could buy a seduction kit online.

That's it. Have fun. You might even think of some games on your own. The important thing to remember is that both parties have fun and enjoy each other.

# Chapter 8: The Secrets to a Great Massage

We have gone over the art of the tantric massage, but if you don't want to take things to that extreme yet, you can still give your partner a simple massage. These techniques will help to make the simple massage more pleasurable.

In our life, it is very easy to let our emotional distance and stress get in the way of having a healthy relationship with our significant other. An erotic massage can help to create physical closeness and intimacy while helping to relieve stress and letting them get into the mood for sex.

When you add in erotic massage to your relationships, it can help to bring you both closer together emotionally and physically. It does not matter if your partner is always stressed or they aren't feeling inspired; an erotic massage can be exactly what you need to explore brand new levels of sexual bliss.

## Three Important Areas of Erotic Massage

For you to get all the benefits of an erotic massage, let's look at the essential elements and how to use them.

- Environment

Setting the scene is very important because the environment could easily break or make the experience. This doesn't have to be time-consuming or expensive. If you incorporate the three things below, you will be doing fine.

First thing, you need to create an environment that doesn't have any distractions. Get any laptops, tablets, or phones out of the room you are going to be in. Unplug the television and cover up any devices that have harsh displays. You will also want something comfortable for them to lay on, and you can use some aromatherapy.

- Mindset

Before the massage, you need to ask yourself:

- How could I make their experience as enjoyable and relaxing as possible?

- How can I stay focused through the whole massage?

- How could I communicate with them to give them the most pleasure?

- What should I look for in their responses or reactions?

How you answer these questions could help you keep the right mindset throughout the entire session. It might take you some time to figure this out; it is going to be worth it to give your partner an erotic and relaxing experience they deserve.

- Technique

Even though the mindset and environment are needed for an erotic massage, it wouldn't be a massage without a technique.

There are some techniques that you can use during the massage:

o Effleurage

At the start of any massage, you should begin with gentle and light touches. These are called effleurage. The reasoning behind this is to get their blood circulating and get them prepared for the massage.

Use the palm of your hand and start with a gentle touch. You can do this in any pattern you want. Circular motions are the most common. They will cover the most area. Make sure you keep the pressure constant and make sure you pay the same attention to all areas of their body.

o Kneading

This is the most common technique that is used during the massage. It is easy to learn how to do.

Use your fingertips and thumb, take the muscle tissue between them, and squeeze at different intervals. This is great for large muscles of the buttocks, upper arms, and thighs.

o Friction

This is normally associated with deep tissue massages. This technique could be used when you need to work out tight kinks. Using your fingertips and thumb, put some gentle pressure on the knot and work it slowly in a circle.

When the knot starts giving away to the pressure, add more pressure while making sure your partner doesn't feel any discomfort.

To lighten the hurts but feels good feelings that are associated with this technique, you can change up the pressure during the session to give your significant other some time to recuperate every once in a while.

o   Stretching

If your significant other has some stubborn areas of stress with knots, stretching could give them the best relief. This technique uses manual manipulation on your significant other's joints. You could rotate their ankles and wrists gently, bend and stretch their elbows and knees, and keep working on getting their limbs as loose and free as you possibly can without using force.

o   Percussion

The chopping motions that are used with this technique might not seem erotic at all, but this could be a fun way to experiment and see how each other likes it.

There are different ways to do this technique. You could use the side of your hands to make a fast chopping motion to the upper back and things. You could use your fingertips to tap out any knots or kinks your find in their lower back, face, and neck. Percussion is useful to have in your massage arsenal.

## The Science of An Erotic Massage

If you have never really entered the world massage, then you may be asking yourself how a simple massage can provide you with the benefits that we went over in the tantric massage chapter. This is a fair question. Humans are sensory-seeking creatures. From a very young age, humans are taught that touch is something we want and is good. We touch people in order to give and receive comfort, show signs of solidarity, and provide warmth.

We touch our partners to show them that we care about them and to provide them with satisfaction and joy. This means that massage can be an easy way to show your significant other that you care about them and their wellbeing. Also, think about the fact that there are certain levels of openness and trust that comes along with a sensual massage.

Very few women are going to be open to receiving an erotic massage from a man if there isn't some level of trust between them, as this contributes to the positive feelings and benefits of an erotic massage.

There are many different processes that the body undergoes when it receives a massage. Some of these processes, like the relaxation of muscles, are local. Others, like the release of endorphins, affects the entire body. But what the exact mechanisms behind the things that are happening?

There are various theories among experts. Some researchers and scientists believe that physical touch through massage session is able to improve circulation. This will, in turn, increase how much oxygen gets delivered to the muscle and will help to improve the healing process. Others believe that massages engage the lymphatic system.

This will help to remove waste from the knotted area and will improve muscle movement and healing. Still, there are those that believe all of the benefits of massage are based in the nervous system. Touch causes an electric sensation that travels from the original point of touch all the way to the brain, which will release endorphins and other happy chemicals. So which one of these theories is right?

Right now, there aren't any right or wrong answers. It is possible that none of the above are correct, or they all could be. But whatever the exact reason is for those "good" feelings, there is no arguing with the scientific research that backs the benefits that come with a massage.

From lowering depression and anxiety levels to control inflammation following physical activities, massage has certainly shown that it provides many benefits to those who undergo treatment.

## Eroticism and Massage

After you have a good understanding of how massage works and all of the benefits it provides, it is easy to see how erotic massage came to be. After all, when you mix two things that help to make you feel, which in this case is sex and massage, it makes sense that those good feelings are going to be amplified.

Erotic massage, though, is not all about sexual pleasure. Instead, there are two ways to pleasure your partner during an erotic massage session. Of course, sexual pleasure is one of these two sources. But, the other pleasure source is from the actual massage.

The orgasm should be seen as a by-product of your massage session, but it should not be the ultimate goal. As you move your hands over their body, your partner is going to feel more relaxed. The tension is going to leave their body, ever so slowly, until all of their muscles are loose and relaxed. This is the reason why climax becomes more likely. As they relax, so will their inhibitions.

With an erotic massage, your partner is going to slowly lose their signs of self-consciousness, anxiety, and fear. This is the magic of an erotic massage.

## Targeted Massage Combinations

Knowing the massage techniques outlined above is a great start, but to make sure that your partner receives the satisfaction they deserve, it is important that you know the areas of the body that you should target and in which manner. The techniques can defiantly be used from head to toe, but sometimes a routine that includes targeted combinations of different body parts can provide more satisfaction.

The orgasm is the greatest possible release that a person can experience. While orgasms can vary in intensity and length, with the right massage routine, you can help to increase the strength of the orgasm. That's what this targeted massage routine is going to help you do.

Begin by having your partner lay flat on their back on a comfortable surface, be it bed, table, or floor. You will start with an entire body once over. This is basically a quick rundown of the more thorough routine you will be doing, but it will help to get the blood pumping. With only your fingertips, start at their forehead. Grave the side of the face with both hands and then slowly move your way down to their neck and chest.

Do not touch their nipples, but do lightly touch around the chest or breasts and then down the sides of their torso. Once you get to their hips, you are going to start to branch out with one hand on one leg and the other hand on the other leg.

Simultaneously move your way down their legs. Remember that you should keep your touches light and feathery, and then trace your way back up a little ways and then back down again. Make sure you notice your partner's cues during this once over so that you can be a good idea of where their most sensitive areas are.

Once you have finished the once over, move back up to their neck. You will work your way down their body once more, but this time you will be spending time kneading the tight kinks and knots out of their body, but you should also add in some light touches to excite and arouse them. You can also use some of the other techniques that we discussed early in the chapter, like stretching. Pay attention to how your partner responds to the different methods.

Since this massage is meant to increase the orgasm, you will want to maximize the touches to the pubic region you make to help excite them. If you are massaging a woman, this does not mean you have to spend a bunch of time on her clitoris. Instead, use light pressure just above the pubic bone. Run your fingers over their stomach and stop at the very top of the public bone right above the hips but just below their belly button.

With the palm of your non-dominant hand, press down slightly. Make sure that your partner isn't uncomfortable. With the dominant hand, slowly work across their genitals, gently grazing across the sensitive areas.

When massaging a woman, feel free to insert your middle and ring fingers into her vagina at this point and press the palm of that hand up against the clitoris. As you move your entire hand up and down, the middle and ring fingers will be hitting the g-spot, and the palm will be rubbing the clitoris. When massaging a man, you can start stroking him.

As you notice them getting closer to climax, you can press down onto the pubic bone a bit more firmly and increase the intensity of your strokes.

These are only a few of the most common techniques that are used during an erotic massage session. You can experiment with various touches. Just remember to watch your partner and their reactions.

The next time you notice that your partner is feeling stressed out, offer to give them a massage and try out these techniques.

# Chapter 9: Trying Dirty Talk

Dirty talk doesn't have to be complicated, weird, awkward, or creepy. Dan Savage, a popular sex columnist, summed up sex talk with this very simple statement, "Tell 'em what you're going to do, tell 'em what you're doing, tell 'em what you did." Simply put, dirty talk should be straightforward and simple.

While it can be and should be simple, most of us end up freezing up in the moment, and we end up saying something we heard once in a porn, and it will come out sound weird, awkward, unnatural, or very unsexy.

Given how easy dirty talk can go wrong, why do we even want to bother with trying it at all? The simplest answer is that when it is done right and is said by a person that you are attracted to, nothing is sexier than vocal sex. The biggest sex organ is the brain, so it only makes sense that we get turned on by what a person says during a moment of passion. This will also work in reverse. When you say your fantasies and desires that normally get kept to yourself to a rapt audience, it can be a big turn-on.

When you will get to the heart of dirty talk, having good dirty talk can take us out of our regular lives and really put us into the act of sex. While you might be physically feeling what is going on, if your mind is not there, the pleasure reward can fall short. This is the reason why people often fantasize when masturbating. Dirty talk helps us get out of our own heads into the body. The simple sounds and tones can help all of our daily worries melt away and remember how amazing our partner feels.

Now that you know why you should try dirty talk, let's look at how you can make it work.

## Don't Make It Complicated

You shouldn't try to be a porn start right off the bat. Say the things that feel natural, and definitely don't think you need to have some sort of elaborate narrative before you get things going. This isn't some strange Shakespearean monologue that you have to recite, and there is no need to talk every single time. Dirty talk doesn't have to just happen during sex. Picking the right moment to say something like, "I can't wait to feel you inside me," can do the trick.

Think about your senses, if vulgar or profane language isn't something that you typically use, then don't feel like you have to. Chances are, your partner would be turned off if you all of a sudden started using words you have never used before. Your aim should be to be playful, and you should start early. While your partner is at work or picking up some things from the store, drop a few hints about how you want to play.

This helps to build the anticipation of sex. You can easily send a text that says, "I can't stop thinking about tonight…"

## Give Instructions

You have two forms of dirty talk. One form helps to build anticipation for sex, and the other is simply instructional and happens, most of the time, during sex. Giving some direction or instructions can be pretty sexy. You could tell your partner something like, "When you get home, I want you to put on your best lingerie, and then I want you to lay, face down, on the bed, and wait for me to come home and play with you." This combines both forms of dirty talk and can be used to add in some role-playing.

## You Don't Have to Go X-Rated

It is very important that you know how to read your partner when it comes to dirty talk. You should not say things that are really vulgar unless all of the signs point to that. You can easily say things that are way too X-rated and then end up turning your partner off. If this happens, it will likely be embarrassing, but you should be able to recover from it.

## If Things Don't Work Out, Talk About What Went Wrong

If something you say causes nervous laughter, that is fine, but there could be times when what you say can trigger them. They may not know the best way to verbalize why those words hurt them in the moment, but if you feel as if you took things too far, you should make a point of talking to them about it later on.

It will help to make sure that both of you understand that dirty talk carves out an erotic space and that you don't actually feel the way the person is talking. It is all about play. Think about how some people like to be called "daddy," but they aren't interested in incest. Instead, they like the dominance and authority the word gives them.

If you do take it too far, then do your best to correct it. Honor what your partner is into and what they are comfortable with, and talk with them about the things that they don't like. But, you should never make them feel like that owe you an explanation for the things they don't like. If they want to tell you, they will. This is true for you as well.

## Try These Out

So, to make things easier for you, if you really don't know what you should say to your partner, I will provide you with a list of lines that you try using. You will have to fill in the blank on some things, but I think you will get the gist pretty quickly.

1. "Fuck me hard."

2. "I love it when you moan my name."

3. "I want you to use me like a toy."

4. "You taste so good."

5. "I'm going to come for you."

6. "It makes me crazy when you _____."

7. "When I get home, I want you in my favorite skirt with no underwear..."

8. "Yes, please. More."

9. "Right there. Touch my _____."

10. "I've been thinking about what I want to do with you..."

Give some of these a try the next time you want to get your partner in the mood and see how it feels.

# Chapter 10: Orgasm

The orgasm has long been viewed as the peak of sexual excitement. It's a very powerful feeling of pleasure, which involves releasing accumulated erotic tension. While everybody's goal with sex is an orgasm, there isn't a lot now about it. During the last few centuries, theories about the orgasm have changed. For example, experts have only recently started talking about the female orgasm. Many doctors in the 1970s claimed it was perfectly normal for a woman not to experience an orgasm.

Orgasms are able to be defined in several ways with different criteria. Medical professionals talk about physiological changes that happen within the body. Mental health professionals and psychologists talk about cognitive and emotional changes. There isn't a single, overarching definition of the orgasm.

Sex researchers have tried to define orgasms in models of sexual response. While the process for orgasm can differ between people, there are several basic physiological changes that often occur in most incidences. Master and Johnson's Four-Phase Model includes:

- Excitement

- Plateau

- Orgasm

- Resolution

Kaplan came up with his own model, but his is different from most sexual response models because it includes desire. The majority of models don't include non-genital changes. It is important to understand, though, that not every sexual act is preceded by desire. Kaplan's three-stage model is:

- Desire

- Excitement

- Orgasm

## Benefits of Orgasm

A 1997 cohort suggested that men's mortality risk was lowered when they experienced a high number of orgasms than in men who had fewer orgasms. There is also some research that suggests ejaculation can help to reduce the risk of prostate cancer. Researchers found that a man's prostate cancer risk was 20 percent lower in those who ejaculated at least 21 times a month than those who ejaculated only four to seven times a month.

There are a lot of hormones that are released during orgasm, which includes DHEA and oxytocin. There are some studies that suggest these hormones may help protect against heart disease and certain cancers. Oxytocin, along with other endorphins that get released during the female and male orgasm are also relaxants.

## Types of Orgasm

Not surprisingly, since experts haven't come to a consensus in regards to a definition of an orgasm, there are many different types of orgasms. Sigmund Freud stated that immature and young females can only have an orgasm through clitoral stimulation while mature women are able to have an orgasm through vaginal stimulation. We will go over a few of those types.

- Pressure orgasms – this orgasm comes from indirect stimulation of applied pressure. This is a type of self-simulation that is common in young people.

- Tension orgasms – this is a common type of orgasm. It is created through direct stimulation, often when the muscles and body are tense.

- Blended or combination orgasm – these are a variety of orgasmic experiences that blend together.

- Relaxation orgasms – this orgasm comes from deep relaxation through sexual stimulation.

- Multiple orgasms – these are a series of orgasms that happen over a short period of time.

There are actually a few orgasms that both Dodson and Freud discounted, but there are others who believe they are real. For example:

- G-spot orgasms – this is an orgasm that is caused by the stimulation of an erotic zone inside the vagina through penetrative intercourse, which feels very different from orgasms caused by other forms of stimulation.

- Fantasy orgasm – these are orgasms that result from mental stimulation.

## The Female Orgasm

Men and women go through similar yet different physiological processes when experiencing an orgasm. Here we will talk about the process of the female orgasm following the Masters and Johnson Four-Phase Model.

1. Excitement

When a woman is psychologically or physically stimulated, the blood vessels in her genitals will dilate. This increased blood flow will make the vulva swell, and fluid will pass through the vaginal walls. This makes the vulva wet and swollen. Internally, the vagina expands at the top. Breathing and heart rate will quicken, and her blood pressure will rise. The blood vessel dilations can cause a woman to look flushed, especially on her chest and neck.

2. Plateau

As the blood flows to the lower vaginal area, it will reach a limit and turn firm. Breasts can also increase in size by 25 percent and increase the blood to the areola, which makes the nipples look less erect. The clitoris will then pull back against the pubic bone, which makes it look like it has disappeared.

3. Orgasm

The genital muscles will experience rhythmic contractions that are about 0.8 seconds apart. For women, their orgasms last longer at about 13 to 51 seconds. Since women don't have a recovery period, they can continue to experience orgasms if they are stimulated again.

4. Resolution

The body will slowly return back to its previous state, with a reduction in breathing, pulse rate, and swelling.

The Male Orgasm

1. Excitement

When a man experiences psychological or physical stimulation, he gets an erection. Blood flow has increased in the corpora, which is the tissue that runs through the penis, which causes the penis to grow and become hard. The testicles will draw up as the scrotum tightens.

2. Plateau

With the increased blood flow, the testicles and glans will increase in size. The buttock and thigh muscles will tense, the pulse quickens, blood pressure rises, and breathing increases.

3. Orgasm

Semen, which is a mixture of 95 percent fluid and 5 percent sperm, is forced through the urethra by contractions in the pelvic floor, vas deferens, seminal vesicles, and prostate gland. These contractions also cause the semen to be forced out of the penis, causing ejaculation. Orgasm for a man tends to last for ten to 30 seconds.

4. Resolution

The man is now in the recovery phase, where he can't have any more orgasms. This is what is called a refractory period, and how long it lasts varies between men. It could be a few minutes to a few days and tends to become longer the older the man becomes. At this point, the testicles and penis return o their original size. Their pulse and breathing will be fast.

## Multiple Orgasms

People find the idea of multiple orgasms intriguing and fro good reason. It is perfectly normal to want to experience one right after the other, as well as simply tapping out after the first. Here, we will go over why the female body is designed to experience multiple orgasms, and strategies to make them more likely to happen.

Having multiple orgasms doesn't necessarily mean that you have another orgasm right after your first one without a moment's rest, but you can do that. Multiple orgasms simply mean that you have several orgasms during a single sexual encounter.

In order to experience multiple orgasms, it will require some experimentation on your part. After you have your first, you will need to figure out what can make it happen again. If you find that your clitoris is so sensitive that you can't touch it, use the rest of your body. Try out different forms of stimulation. This could be playing with your breasts or getting your partner to kiss everything except the clitoris. The main point is to continue the arousal in whatever way works for you. Continue this for however long you want, and you can always check back in with the clitoris to see if some of the sensitivity has gone away.

That being said, sometimes stimulating the sensitive clitoris could be the ticket. There are some women who say continuing to run the clitoris gives them the chance to embrace what seems like unbearable overstimulation, which can result in more orgasms. It all depends on what you are able to handle. If you like oversensitivity, then do it. If it hurts or doesn't seem to be creating a pleasurable feeling, stop touching the clitoris to try to have more orgasms.

You can also use Kegal exercises to help extend your orgasms. As you reach your first orgasm, push your hand over your vulva and pulse it between orgasm contractions as you squeeze your thighs. Doing this can intensify and increase the orgasmic contraction and bring you into another orgasm.

You also need to make sure that you breathe during the entire experience. There are some people who will unconsciously hold their breath as the orgasm builds, but concentrating can help. When you reach an orgasm, breathe purposefully, slowly, and deeply while contracting your pelvic floor muscles. This breath work can lead to multiples for some people.

These tips are a great place to start, but don't get upset if they don't work the first time. It takes practice and learning your body.

# Chapter 11: Female Ejaculation

Ejaculation has been described as a powerful experience that is only associated with male sexuality and penises. What most people don't realize is that it is possible for a female to ejaculate from the vagina or vulva. This could happen after, during, or even before sex and with or without an orgasm. Since there is a lot more knowledge about women and people, who were assigned the female persona at birth do possess sexuality. We aren't just passive sex objects. We are more aware and open about our sexual appetites, desires, and biology. Squirting is only one small part of it.

## What Is It?

While having sex, some people who have vulvas will experience an involuntary release of fluids. This is what is known as female ejaculation or, as some people call it, squirting. Even though everyone who has a vulva identifies themselves as a female, and everybody who identifies as a female won't have a vulva.

"Squirting" has gotten more attention recently because more people are talking about it. There is more accurate information about the sexual reality of people who were assigned the gender of female. Their bodies are still thought of as being a mystery or myth. Squirting is often thought of as something to try to reach or just a part of being completely liberated sexually. This puts a lot of unnecessary pressure on women.

Some people think that squirting is just a party trick that specific people have to perform. But that doesn't make anyone feel empowered. What about people who identify outside the gender norms? How can we talk about female ejaculation?

## Squirting History

It seems as if ejaculation has been around for a long time. During 2010, Joanna Korda and her associates looked through numerous ancient literary texts and found many references about sexual fluids being ejaculated.

In the ancient India text the *Kama Sutra*, they talk about "female semen that falls constantly." In a Taoist text written during the 300x called *Secret Instructions Concerning the Jade Chamber*, they talk about the difference between "the genitals transmitting fluid" and a slippery vagina. Joanna Korda and her conspirators concluded that this could easily be considered to be female ejaculation.

Most people wouldn't even consider it to be literature. They see it as pornography. Pornography is a normal way for anyone to learn about sex now. We checked out one popular porn side called Pornhub and found that some of the most popular videos were about squirting. The popularity of squirting increased a lot between the years 2013 and 2015. It still remains as some of their top 20 videos.

According to their data, women search for squirting videos 44 percent more than men do. As people age, the popularity of squirting will decrease.

People from Slovakia, Venezuela, Columbia, Vietnam, and South Africa will search for squirting videos when compared to other countries. In America, people from Wyoming, Montana, Utah, and Nebraska are more interested in squirting videos as compared to people from New Jersey, Maryland, California, and New York.

Most people who are assigned the female gender only experience something like a trickle rather than the large gushes that you see in videos. In fact, most people don't even realize it happened. Just like not squirting or squirting is "better," there isn't a right or wrong way when ejaculating.

## What Is the Fluid That Gets Ejaculated?

Just because squirting videos are popular doesn't mean that it is accepted everywhere. During 2014, any pornography depicting female ejaculation was banned in Europe. This ban has been met with a lot of protests because it implies that ejaculating from the vulva or vagina is perverted while ejaculating from a penis is totally normal.

Censors couldn't see the difference between urination and female ejaculation. They consider urination to be and "obscene" act.

Scientists haven't agreed on what exactly is in the fluid of the female ejaculation. Even though it still isn't clear, female ejaculation fluid has shown to contain some urine, and it contains other fluids, too.

Dr. Amy Gilliland, a sex researcher, did a study in 2009 along with Doula and found that studies that have been done on female ejaculation noticed those studies didn't include how the people felt about the account.

Most of the participants reported that large amounts of fluid were released during their orgasm. Some stated there was enough that it sprayed walls, soaked the bed, and scared their partners.

Gilliland saw that some women who felt shameful about their ejaculation learned to feel more positive about their ejaculation later on in life once they heard other people's positive feedback, other's experiences, and learned more about female ejaculation.

# Chapter 12: Best Sex Positions for Him

The tantric and kama sutra sex positions that we will talk about in this chapter are great for everyone involved, but it focuses on what will feel the best for him. While this chapter and the next will use the pronouns of he and she, this doesn't mean same-sex couples can't try these positions. They are adaptable to any couple who would like to try them.

## Rock-a-Bye Booty

This one can be a bit tricky for people who aren't exactly flexible.

- Begin with the man on his back, and the lady slowly straddles him.

- Once he has penetrated her, he will lift his torso up, and she will position herself so that they are facing each other.

- Both will wrap their legs tightly around each other's buttocks. Both will link their elbows under the other's knees and bring them up so that they are at chest level.

This position will require a rocking motion since thrusting isn't possible in this position. The woman can squeeze her pelvic floor muscles to provide him with a stronger sensation.

# Passion Pretzel (Blooming Orchid)

In the scheme of things, this position is fairly simple. If you or your partner have bad knees, then you may want to make sure you have cushions for your knees to rest on.

- To get into this position, start by kneeling face-to-face.

- Then you will both place the opposite foot flat on the floor and inch closer until your genitals reach each other.

- You both place your weight on your planted foot, and you both lunge back and forth.

This position places you in equal positions, and you share the reins. Everybody's arms are free to do as they will, as well. This will be a slow grind and not a lot of in-and-out action.

## The G-Force

This is a fairly simple move that almost anybody can do. The man will have reins in this one.

- She lays down and pulls her knees as far into her chest as she can.

- He will kneel in front of her and grab hold of her feet and then thrusts into her.

- He can then bring her feet up to his chest. The woman will only have her upper back on the bed or floor.

## Baby Got Back

For this one:

- The man will kneel and then sit back on his heels.

- The woman keeps her back to him and lowers herself onto his penis, either in a squat or plie. Her feet should be planted on either side of him.

- She places her hands on her thighs to help her keep her balance. He can also hold her rear to help with support.

- She slowly moves up and down, and she can nest all the way into his lap. She controls the movement with this position.

## Tub Tangle

This one will take bath time to a whole new level.

- He will sit reclined in the tub, and she will straddle his lap while facing him.

- Once he is inside of her, he will move his torso up so that they are more face-to-face.

- They will both wrap their legs around one another's backs and link their elbows under the other's knees to pull them up to chest level.

This will require slight rocking instead of thrusting.

## Lap Dance

For this one, you are going to need a tall-backed chair that you have padded with some pillows to make things more comfortable.

- He will sit down in the chair.

- She will face him and straddle him, sliding him inside of her, and then lean back a bit. She should rest her hands on his knees.

- One at a time, she will bring her legs up so that her ankles are resting on his shoulders.

- She will then move her buttocks back and forth, and at whatever speed she likes.

This will take some balance power on the woman's part.

## The Milk and Water Embrace

This is great for all types of people.

- He sits down on the bed, a short stool, or chair.

- She then sits down on him, with her back to him.

- She then controls the thrusting.

This leaves all hands free to do as they will.

## Torrid Tidal Wave

This is great for an intense make-out session.

- He will lay on his back, keeping his legs together.

- She will straddle his penis and then move to lay stretched out on top of him, pelvises aligned.

- She will lift up her torso so that she is resting on her hands.

- The slightest movements will provide pleasing friction.

## The Tug of Love

For this position:

- He will lay down first with his legs wide open.

- She will down on top of him and allow him to enter her. Her legs should be on either side of him stretched out in front of her.

- Then she will lean back onto the bed.

- Once both are laying down, he will grab her hands and gently pull them to move her.

This is great for couples who have a foot fetish.

## Life Raft

This is designed for sex in the water. You will need a pool and an inflatable pool bed.

- She will position herself on the pool bed on her stomach. Her vagina should be in the middle of the bed.

- He stands behind her with her legs wrapped around his hips. He should not push downwards. He enters and starts thrusting.

The important thing is to make sure the vagina stays out of the water because the water, especially if it is chlorinated, can dry things out.

## Brute

This is a very male dominant position.

- She will lay down and pull her knees to her chest.

- He will stand with his back to her, straddling her hips.

- He then squats down and slowly enters her and continues to move slightly up and down.

The man needs to be very careful not to hurt himself.

## Piston

This can be quite a tiring position.

- Both are standing and facing each other.

- He will lift her off the ground, placing his arms under her butt and thighs.

- Having a bed or sofa behind him will allow her to let her legs rest on it to help take some weight off of him.

- He will then "piston" himself up and down.

This might be easier to get into if he starts out sitting on a bed or sofa.

## Missionary

This is a common one and one you have already performed, but it is a very intimate position.

- She will be on her back with her legs open.

- He will rest on his elbows as he thrusts in and out.

## Helicopter

For this, the penis will need to be slightly flexible. Not every man will be able to do this. Basically, if you are standing, you should be able to push your erect penis down towards the ground comfortably before trying this.

- She will begin by laying on her stomach, with her legs straight and wide.

- He will then lay down on his stomach, facing the opposite direction, legs straight and wide.

- He will back into her until his thighs are over hers, and he can push his penis into her. He can then slowly and carefully thrust in and out of her.

## Face to Face

This is great when you want to be intimate. Plus, it doesn't take a lot of effort.

- She will need to be sitting on the edge of a sofa, bed, or any other surface that is about 12 to 20 inches off the ground.

- He will kneel in front of her.

- She can drop herself slightly over the edge to help line things up.

- He can grab hold of her legs or waist when he starts to thrust.

## Book Ends

Some couples struggle with this one, so you will need to experiment.

- Both will begin on their knees facing each other.

- He will spread his knees so that he can be closer to the bed while she will remain tall.

- Once he has lowered himself so that he is in line with her, he can slip his penis inside.

- If comfortable, he can move his knees back together.

## Jellyfish

This can be a difficult position. It requires some strength and balance for both people.

- He starts by kneeling in the bed, his butt resting on his ankles.

- She will straddle him, squatting so he can enter.

- Both will wrap their arms around one another.

You will be doing more of a grinding motion rather than thrusting.

## Hang Loose

This is a variation of missionary.

You will do the same thing you did for missionary, except this time, you will be on the edge of the bed so that her head can hang over the edge.

## Big Dipper

This is a tiring sex position, so don't plan on being here too long. You will need a sturdy chair that faces your sofa or bed.

- He will position himself so that he isn't quite sitting in the chair, with his hands resting on the chair and his feet on the bed or sofa. He will be completely elevated off the ground. He will look like he is going to do a tricep dip.

- She will then straddle his as she is facing him, but she should not place any weight on him.

- He will then lower himself and push himself back up, moving in and out of her.

## Reverse Missionary

This is another one that will require some penis flexibility.

- She will start by laying down with her legs spread apart.

- He will lay down on top of her but facing her feet. His legs should rest on either side of her.

- He will slowly push his penis into her.

Any position that requires him to move his penis backward needs to be done carefully and the partner should never pull on the penis. It is very easy to hurt the suspensory ligaments.

## Ballerina Sex Position

This one will require the woman to be flexible to do this comfortably.

- Both will start by standing and facing each other.

- She will raise one leg up until it rests on his shoulder as she balances on the other.

- The raised leg will be pretty much straight so that he can get as close as possible.

- He can wrap his arms around her as he starts thrusting.

## Screw

This is a simple position that anybody can do.

- She will start by lying down on her side.

- He will position himself behind her legs and place his hands on either side of her torso.

- She will turn her upper body to face him as he starts penetrating her.

## Stand and Carry

This is a standing position that does not use a couch, bed, or wall.

- She starts off lying down, and he will lean over her. She wraps her arms around his neck and her legs around his waist once he enters you.

- He then wraps his arms around her and brings her to a standing position. He can grab her butt to help move her up and down.

## Bent Spoon

This isn't one of the most popular sex positions, but it is great if you want to shake things up.

- The man will lay on his back, and she will lay on top of him, back to his chest.

- He will then enter her.

- She will then spread arms out to help keep her steady, and he will spread his legs to keep his balance.

- Once ready, she will bring her knees up to her chest and rest her feet on his knees for support.

## X Marks the Spot

This is another variation of the missionary positions.

- She will start by laying in her back with the man on top.

- Hence the name, their bodies will make an X.

This might be a bit tricky at first, and possibly awkward, but once you get into it, it should get easier.

## Italian Chandelier

This position is very submissive for the woman and gives the man a lot of power. It is super easy to move from missionary to the Italian Chandelier.

- Begin by getting into a regular missionary sex position.

- He will then come up on his knees, bringing them closer to the woman, which should force her legs apart.

- He then wraps his hands under her hips and butt and then lifts them up.

- She will help out by planting her feet on the bed. The goal is to have her hips and waist pushed into the air.

## Down Stroke

There is a lot of stimulation for both people with this move.

- She will lay on her back close to the edge of the sofa or bed and raise her legs into the air so that they are pointed towards the ceiling.

- He will stand in front of her and grab her legs, pulling her toward him so he can enter her.

- Once he has her lifted towards him, he will lift her waist off the bed so that only her shoulders and upper back are touching the bed.

## Exposed Eagle

This is one of the hardest Kama sutra positions we will discuss in the book. It requires a lot of strength and flexibility.

- The easiest way to start is to begin in cowgirl position. She will straddle and face him with her knees on either side.

- She will then lay backward until her back in on his knees and thighs. He has the option of raising his knees if she can't bend all the way backward.

- He will then raise his upper body so that he is in a more seated position.

- He can support himself by placing his arms behind him, or he can wrap them around her back.

## Bended Knee

This is an easier version of the ballerina.

- Both will start out on their knees facing each other—they need to be close.

- He stays on one knee and lifts the other up and out to plant his foot.

- She will then lift the leg in front of his raised nee and rest her leg over his.

- He can then enter and begin thrusting.

## Acrobat

This is a variation of the reverse cowgirl.

- He will begin by lying on his back, and then she will straddle him, facing away from him.

- She will stay on her knees and will then lay back onto him.

## Viennese Oyster

This is a more complicated position that will require some flexibility.

- She will start on her back and grab her legs, pulling them apart and back.

- She will want to get her legs so far back that they are touching or almost touching the bed on either side of her. She can then wrap her arms around her legs.

- He can then enter. He could also hold her legs back.

## Crab

This is another one that should only be done if he has a great deal of penile flexibility because she will be bending the penis back quite a bit when she sits on him.

- Begin by getting into a cowgirl position.

- She will then move her feet so that they are planted on either side of his shoulders.

- She then bends back, slightly, supporting herself on her hands.

This position should not be used during rough sex because it could damage the penis.

## Bouncing Spoons

This is a super simple position that any couple can do.

- He will sit upright in bed with his back supported against the wall or headboard. His legs should be relatively straight out in front of him.

- She will stand over him, back to him, her feet positioned on either side of his legs.

- She will then move down onto her knees and sit back onto him, guiding his penis inside of her.

- She can then lean back so that she is rested against his chest.

## Side Ride

This is another variation of the cowgirl position and is super easy to do.

- He will begin by lying down with his knees bent slightly so that his feet are flat on the bed to give him thrusting leverage.

- She will then sit on his lap, letting him enter her. Instead of having her back to him or facing him, she will sit sideways. This means she will face left or right.

## Deep Impact

Hence the name, this position will allow for deep penetration. This is great for rough, passionate sex.

- She will lay down and point her legs towards the ceiling.

- He will be position on his knees, facing her.

- She will rest her legs against her shoulders.

- He then grabs her thighs and holds her tight as he thrusts.

## Twister

This is definitely an "exotic" sex position.

- She will start by lying down her side. For this example, we will use the right side.

- He will then lay down on his right side. His head will be at her feet and her head at his feet.

- They will both bend their left knees and raise them up to the ceiling.

- She will lean forward and push her body through the newly created gap so that his leg is now over her waist. She should not be lying on his right leg.

- He will be sandwiched between her legs with her left legs over his waist.

- He should now be able to start thrusting.

## See Saw

This is fun but can be quickly tiring. This is also a very unique position.

- He will sit down on the bed.

- She will sit in his lap, facing him.

- She should spread her legs wide so that she can get comfortable.

- She can then start to lean back, and either rest her hands on his shoulders or place them behind her.

You can either move up and down or grind on each other.

## Intersection

This position will require you to form a cross with your bodies.

- Both will start out lying on their sides. She will have her head at one end and her feet at the other. He will lay across the bed.

- She will open her legs so that he can lay down on top of the lower one and penetrate her.

## Doggy Style

This is a position that everybody knows and can do.

- She starts on her hands and knees with her legs spread apart.

- He is positioned behind her on his knees and enters from behind.

## Sockets

This is a variation of scissoring.

- She starts by lying on her back with her legs spread wide.

- She will then bend her knees and plant her feet so that she can lift her lower back and waist off of the bed.

- He will then lay on his side at the other end of the bed.

- He should move down towards her in order to enter her. As he does so, he will slide his leg on hers. If he is on his right side, his right leg will move under her left leg and will move his left leg over her left leg. If he is on his left, he will do the opposite.

This is another position where his penis will need to be flexible.

## Turtle

This is a variation of doggy and will require a bit more flexibility.

- She will begin by getting into the doggy position by resting on her knees.

- She will lower herself down so that she is resting on her ankles.

- Then she will lean as far forward as she can. She can reach behind and grab hold of her legs to help her lean further forward.

- He will then be on his knees behind her, penetrating her.

## Lazy Wheelbarrow

While this may have lazy in the name, it still takes a lot of effort.

- He will start by sitting on a sofa with his legs together.

- She then sits down on him, facing away, with her legs together.

- She will start to lean forward as far as she can so that she can place her hands on the floor. Her stomach will be resting on her thighs.

## Fire Hydrant

This is another doggy style variation.

- Both will get into a regular doggy style position.

- His knees should be positioned inside of hers.

- He will then start to lift one of his legs up and forwards so that his foot is planted at her side.

- The leg he moved will be under her leg so that her thigh will be resting on his thigh. The goal is to look like a dog peeing on a fire hydrant.

# Chapter 13: Best Sex Positions for Her

The goal for these positions isn't to have an earth-shattering orgasm. The journey of lovemaking is about becoming one, being orgasmic, moving, connecting, feeling, and breathing with your partner. When you learn to explore your sexuality while being conscious of everything around you and you learn how to harness its power to experience a profound connection with other humans, you will transcend the need for specific techniques and just get into the flow. This flow will move into every area of your life.

## Yab Yum

For this position:

- The guy is going to sit either on a bed or any other flat surface. He will fold his legs in the position of the half lotus. If this is too uncomfortable for him, have him sit on the edge of the bed or a chair and allow his legs to dangle.

- The woman is going to sit on his lap. Her legs will straddle his. She needs to wrap her legs around his waist. If this isn't comfortable for her, she can place a pillow under her bottom. If you are sitting in a chair, her legs could just dangle over his.

- She is going to raise herself up so she can put his penis inside her vagina. It doesn't matter whether it is hard or soft; either one is fine.

- Place your upper bodies against each other to create more skin on skin sensation. You can wrap your arms around one another.

- When you feel the time is right, you can begin to rock back and forth and let your bodies do the rest.

## "Fitting On Of the Sock" or "The Rolling Tickle"

These are actually two different positions, but they blend together great and are great if you aren't very flexible.

- The woman will lay down on her back with her head resting on a pillow.

- The man is going to kneel down between her legs. He will sit back on his heels. If he needs to support his knees, he can put a pillow between his heels and butt.

- The woman is going to place her legs across the man's legs.

- The man is going to place his penis along the length of the woman's vulva. He will rock back and forth to stimulate the vulva. He uses his hands to stimulate her other erogenous zones.

- Once the woman is extremely excited and well lubricated, the man can place his penis inside her vagina.

- The woman is going to raise her pelvis up to meet him. Make sure you find your rhythm.

- If the woman is fairly flexible, she can bring her knees up to her chest.

- The man will be able to penetrate her very deeply while she is rolling her things down and up. If she needs help or support, he can place his hands under her bottom.

## Congress of a Cow

For this position:

- The woman is going to bend forward at the waist while keeping her feet and hands on the floor

- The man will come up behind her and penetrate her.

- All the woman has to do is keep her balance while he thrusts away.

## Yawning

- The woman is going to lay down on her back.

- The man is going to kneel in between her legs.

- The woman will spread her legs as wide as possible on either side of the man's waist. She will lift her legs as high as she possibly can. To alternate the sensations, she can try moving her legs up and down.

- Since you are both supported on the floor or bed, this is a great position to let your hand wander all over each other's bodies.

## Tripod

- Both the man and woman will stand facing each other.

- The man is going to put one hand under one of her knees and bring it off the floor. You have now become a tripod.

- The man will now penetrate the woman.

- This works best if both parties are about the same height.

## Launch Pad

- The woman is going to lay down on her back.

- The man will penetrate her while staying on his knees and facing her.

- The woman will lift her legs up and bring her knees into her chest. She can rest her feet on his chest if she would like.

- The man can lean over her while she raises her hips so he can penetrate her deeply.

## Coital Alignment Technique

- The woman is going to lay down on her back with her legs spread open.

- The man is going to place himself in between her legs and penetrate her. This is just like performing a normal missionary position.

- Rather than him beginning to thrust in and out, he is going to move forward over her body. This changes the angle of his penis. His penis is now going to point down and will be more in contact with her vagina's back wall.

- While the man is in this position, his pubic bone and possibly penis will be in constant contact with the woman's clitoris.

- The woman doesn't need to just lay there. She can move to keep her clitoris in constant contact with his penis and pubic bone.

- The woman can also wrap her legs around his back and pull him farther into her vagina.

- The woman will get more out of this position if she can get a rhythm going with her man.

## Swan Sport

- The man is going to lay down on the bed or floor on his back.

- The woman will sit on top of the man while facing his feet. She is going to place her feet on top of his thighs.

- She now has the opportunity to go as fast or slow as she would like.

- She needs to be able to keep her balance while sitting on her man.

- The man can help her keep her balance by holding onto her waist.

## Upavitika

- The woman lays down on the floor or bed with her knees bent and feet on the bed.

- The man kneels between her legs and penetrates her.

- Once she has been penetrated, he can straighten his legs out.

- The woman will bring one foot up and place it over his heart.

- She gets to control the situation with her foot over his heart.

## The Mastery

- The man is going to sit on the sofa or side of the bed with his feet flat on the floor. He needs to have his butt and thighs on the bed.

- The woman will either kneel down or squat on his lap.

- The woman can then wrap their arms around his neck.

- Help him penetrate you. Once he is firmly inside you, you can lift yourself up and down on top of him, and he can thrust into you.

- You might find it easier to just rock back and forth or grind against him.

- This position puts the woman in power since she is on top. She can find the rhythm she lays to bring both of you to orgasm.

- Since you are facing each other, you get to kiss and fondle each other.

- To change things up, you can place your hands on his knees and lean back a bit. Just be careful.

## Pearly Gates

- The man is going to lay down on his back. He needs to bend his knees with his feet on the bed.

- The woman is going to lay down on top of the man. The woman's head will be to the side and above his.

- The man will now penetrate the woman while in this position.

- If you have problems keeping your balance, spread your legs, and keep them bent, so your feet are on the bed. You could also spread out your arms to help you balance, too.

- The man can wrap his arms around the woman's chest or waist to help keep them balance while playing with her breasts.

- When the woman has her balance, she will be able to thrust back and forth on his penis while he thrusts up into her.

- Since his mouth is right by her ear, he can talk dirty to her or nibble on her neck and ear.

## Pretzel

- The woman is going to lay down on her side with the leg against the bed straight and the leg on top crooked out just slightly.

- The woman will need to raise her top leg slightly toward her chest and place the arm on top either in front of her or behind her. Just make sure the arms are very comfortable.

- The man is going to come in on his knees and straddle the woman's straight leg while remaining on his knees. Once he has penetrated her, he will keep his torso upright while thrusting into the woman.

- The woman won't be able to do much in this position, so she is at the mercy of her victor.

## The Wheel Barrow

- The woman is going to bend forward at the waist with her hands and feet on the floor.

- The man will come up behind the woman and penetrate her from behind. Once he has penetrated her, he can lift one or both feet off the ground. Again this depends on how strong each of you are.

- The woman's hands and arms might become extremely tired while doing this position. If you have to, you can squeeze your legs together a bit to help you keep your balance.

- While the man is thrusting in and out, the woman just needs to keep her balance. That's pretty much it.

## The Bodyguard

- You are both going to stand up straight.

- You are going to be facing in the same direction.

- The man is going to come up behind the woman and penetrate her.

- If he is taller, he is going to need to bend his knees a bit.

- Once he is inside, he will just thrust in and out, and you can push yourself back into him.

## Asian Cowgirl

- The man is going to lay down on the floor or bed on his back.

- The woman is going to straddle him, but instead of being on her hands and knees like regular cowgirl, she will squat. This means that most of her weight is going to be supported by her feet.

- The woman can use her hands to take the weight off her feet by placing them on the man's chest or beside him on the bed.

## Irish Garden

- To start this position, the man will sit on the bed with his back straight. He needs to keep his legs out in front of him and opened wide. He can bed his knees if it is more comfortable.

- The woman will get on her hands and knees, facing away from him and move backward toward him.

- She will lower herself onto the man by straightening her legs out behind the man make sure there is one leg on each side of his waist.

- Now she can lower her shoulders and head to the bed.

- The woman is responsible for all the movement here since she has the man pinned to the bed.

## The Amazon

- The man will lay down on his back with his legs raised slightly with his knees bent.

- The woman will come in and squat down on him.

- He is going to need to bring his legs closer to his chest, so they don't get in your way.

- Now, sit on his penis and set your pace.

- The man will automatically push you up with his thighs.

## Pump

- The woman is going to stand on a short table, sofa, or bed. Her legs stay bent just a little bit.

- The man will penetrate her from behind while he is standing.

- The woman can place her arms on a wall in front of her if there is one to help her push back against him.

## Superwoman

- The woman is going to lay down on the bed on her stomach. Her arms will be stretched in front of her on the bed.

- The woman's legs need to be hanging off the side of the bed. Her waist should be even with the edge of the bed.

- The man will penetrate her from behind while he is standing and will begin thrusting.

## Bull Dog

- The woman will get on her hands and knees. Then she is going to bring her legs together.

- This man will penetrate her from behind in a slightly squatting position.

- He will put his feet to the outside of her legs. He can keep himself steady by placing his hands on her shoulders or waist.

## Legs on Shoulder

- The woman will lay down on her back and bring her legs up, so they are pointing at the ceiling.

- The man will be positioned on his knees but keeping his back straight. He will penetrate her.

- The woman will rest both her legs on one of his shoulders.

- The man will wrap one arm around her legs while placing the other hand on her stomach.

## Prison Style

- Both the man and woman will be standing and facing in the same direction.

- The man will penetrate the woman from behind.

- The woman will bend at the waist until her chest is parallel to the ground, and she is looking at the floor.

- The woman can spread her legs while the man keeps his closed.

- Now the woman needs to put her arms parallel to her body.

- The man will reach forward and grab her wrists and bring her arms behind her back. He gets to control her by keeping her arms behind her back.

## Burning Man

- The woman is going to face a table or countertop and will bend forward until her stomach is touching the surface. Her feet will stay on the ground.

- The man will come up behind her and penetrate her.

- The woman's legs are going to act as an anchor that will keep you in place. This allows the man to give some intense, hard penetration without falling.

## Praying Mantis

- The woman will lay down on her back with her legs open.

- The man will kneel in front of her pelvis and penetrate her. He will take one of her legs and bring it up slowly so that it points the ceiling.

He can then place it on his shoulder or wrap his arm around it.

## Betty Rocker

- The man will lay down on his back with his legs slightly apart.

- The woman will straddle him while facing away. While she is sitting straight up, she will place his penis inside of her.

- Once he is firmly inside, she will begin leaning forward while supporting herself with her arms on his legs.

- Now the woman will begin to rock back and forth by using her arms and legs. She could also move up and down on his penis.

## Thigh Tide

- The man is going to lay down on his back with his legs straight in front of him.

- He will raise one knee just a bit and put his foot on the bed.

- The woman is going to face away from the man. She is going to place one knee on either side of the man's bent leg while sitting on his penis.

- She will raise herself up and down on him. She can hold on to the man's leg to help keep her balance.

## Fast Fuck

- The man will lay down on his back. His knees will be bent slightly and his feet on the bed.

- The woman will straddle him. She can either stay on her feet or knees. She will lean forward while resting on her elbows or hands. She will position herself, so she is raised above the man just slightly.

- She won't be resting on his crotch.

- The man will begin thrusting into her quickly. It isn't going to be a deep penetration, but it will feel wonderful.

## Jughead

- The man is going to lay down either beside a couch or bed while keeping his back on the floor.

- The man will put his legs up on the bed or sofa.

- The woman will position herself above the man while being on all fours with an arm and a leg on each side of him.

- The man is going to lift his lower back and crotch off the floor so he can penetrate her.

- The woman will sit on his penis and thrust herself back into him. She can thrust as hard as she wants, or he can just push into her while she takes it easy.

## Man Missionary

- The man will lay down on his back with his legs together. He can keep them straight or bend them at the knee.

- The woman will straddle him just like with the cowgirl position.

- The woman will lean forward over the man and rest her hands on his chest or stomach.

- She will then begin rocking back and forth. It is really like the normal Missionary position but reversed.

# Chapter 14: Best Sex Positions To Bring Couples Closer

We've covers positions that are more pleasurable for him and for her, so let's look at some positions that will help to increase the intimacy in the relationship. While those sudden and desperate quickies, but nothing is better than sex that is soulful and rich. This can harness the bonding powers of neurochemistry and science.

## Lotus Blossom

This is also known as the seated wrap-around and will require you and your partner to embrace one another, which is great for gazing romantically into each other's eyes.

This position can be used even if your goal isn't to have sex or orgasm. You can simply sit in their lap and look at each other or make out. To get into the position, one partner will straddle the other as you both sit in a cross-legged position. The person on top will wrap their legs around the bottom of their partner as you two face one another and embrace. The one on the bottom will enter the person on top with a penis or a toy.

## Spooning 69

This position will allow the two of you to give and receive oral play while on your side. You get to have the closeness of spooning while also having the joy of the mouth-to-genital play.

You will both lay on your sides, facing one another but in opposite directions so that your mouth is aligned with your partner's genitals.

## Breakfast Spoons

This is the spooning position but with morning sex. While it may not sound special, having sex in this cuddling position before you have both fully woken up brings something romantic to the relationship.

When your partner enters you from behind in the spooning position, they get the joy of being able to kiss your neck, hold your hands, or provide extra stimulation.

## The Hound

This is an intimate spin on doggy style. This position allows for slow, deep thrusts, as well as quick, shallow thrusts. It is best to start things slowly and then speed it up. Alternate between deep and shallow. With this position, there is a lot more skin-to-skin contact, and all of her other erogenous zones are easily accessible. They can also nibble on the other's neck or ears, whisper dirty phrases.

How to get into this position. Both will start on their knees. The person doing the penetration will have their legs positioned on the outside of their partner and will curl their body around the other person and enter from behind. The one on the bottom will rest on their forearms and will be able to swivel their hips to get into a comfortable position.

## Face-to-Face Standing

Face-to-face sex is great for kissing and intimacy. To get into this position, both partners will stand facing each other. It might be easier if one partner is braced against a wall. The penetrating partner will place themselves between the other's legs. They will penetrate their partner, and if possible, they can lift their partner's legs around their hips.

## Drill

Missionary positions can be one of the most erotic positions because it places you in a face-to-face position. This position takes the standard missionary up a notch.

The woman will start by lying down, just like she would with regular missions. She will then raiser her legs up and wrap them around your partner's waist. She can cross her ankles to help keep her legs around him. This will allow you to grip their partner closer and pull them into her.

## Teaspooning

This is one of the most intimate positions you can try.

He will start out on his knees, spreading them as wide as he comfortably can. She will then get on her knees in front of him, keeping her knees together. He will move closer to her, keeping his legs on either side of hers. He can then enter her, and his arms should be wrapped around her, holding her breasts, or holding her shoulders.

## Sofa Spooning

You will want to make sure you have a comfortable, full-length sofa for this one.

He will lay down on the couch with his back pressed against the back of the couch. She will lay down in front so that they are laying back to chest. He will then enter her and start to slowly thrust with his arms wrapped around her.

This is great for a Netflix and chill moment.

## The Mermaid

For this position, she will lay down face-up at the edge of a counter, desk, or bed. A pillow under her butt may be helpful. She will extend her legs into the air, keeping them together. He will stand in front of her, holding her ankles to keep him stable and allow him to thrust deeper.

## The Sofa Spread-Eagle

This can be tricky if there is a large height difference.

She will start by standing on the edge of the bed, couch, or on two chairs, with her legs spread wide. He will stand on the floor in front of her. She will need to adjust her stance so that he can easily slide until their pelvises meet.

He'll do all the moving on this one, but she can do whatever she wants with her hands.

# Chapter 15: Increasing Male Orgasmic Control

All men are looking to have an intense orgasm and an erection that will last long enough for them to reach orgasm. Reaching an orgasm is simple, but sustaining an erection and enjoying the orgasm will take a little more time and patience. Plus, your partner will thank you for lasting longer. Let's look at how you can control your orgasm and erection.

## Muscle Strength

While having a six-pack might get you noticed, those aren't the muscles that help you during sex. To get the most out of your sexual experience, you need to work on your pubococcygeal muscle. These muscles sit on the floor of your pelvis and control your stream of urine and the muscle spasms that happen when you have an orgasm. This is why sex therapists and doctors recommend that you work on strengthening those muscles so that you don't have premature ejaculations and to improve the orgasm.

Kegel exercises aren't something that only women can do. They can also be used to strengthen the man's PC power. When you are urinating, you can squeeze this muscle to stop the flow of urine. Once you have figure out where the muscle is by doing this, you can squeeze that muscle at any time during the day. Hold the muscle for two seconds and then release. Do this 20 times, three times a day. You will start to hold the muscles for longer intervals. You should never stop with these exercises. Kegel exercises have to be performed on a regular basis in order to keep those muscles strong.

## Edging

Nothing can help you to strengthen your control and erection better than edging, or holding back right before you orgasm. You stop as soon as you feel like you are about to orgasms, rest until you are in control again, and then continue with sex. This can be done until it becomes second nature. This can be practicing during masturbation, and once you are ready to orgasm, you can stop edging.

The best way to edge is, once you stop yourself, don't start again until your breathing is under control, and then wait 30 seconds before you continue on. If you find this does not work, you can also stop ejaculation by squeezing the top of your penis or gently pulling the testicles right when you are about to have an orgasm. Then you will do this all over again. After edging has been mastered, you will be able to have a dry or contractile orgasm. Basically, you will get the same pleasure sensations of an orgasm, but you won't lose the erection. This means that you can have multiple orgasms before you finally finish.

## Stop Masturbating

I understand that I just told you to practice edging while masturbating but hear me out. Masturbating is probably not going to give you and eye-rolling and mind-blowing orgasm for a man at least. The male body releases 400% more prolactin after they have penetrated a vagina than it does after masturbation. Prolactin is the male hormone that makes them feel sexually satisfied. Our evolutionary forces have always rewarded behaviors that are connected with reproduction. Having vaginal-penile sex is something that is passed through our genes.

## Deep Breathing

If you ask a sex therapist the best way to have a full-body orgasm, they are going to tell you that controlled breathing will do it for you. If you make sure that your breathing remains regular and deep, this is going to allow for a more intense arousal to build. The orgasm will remain more satisfying. Breathing to quickly is going to increase your excitement and will ultimately push you over the edge.

Breathing can intensify the male orgasm by taking more oxygen into the arousal process. Shallow breaths in through the nose and deep breaths out through the mouth will help to remove muscular and psychological tension that will help to intensify the orgasm.

## Use the Brain

Orgasms get started in the brain. Our brains are in control of everything and are active in the genitals. Women have a lot of activity within the brain area that is connected to emotions, whereas men only experience brain activity in their secondary somatosensory cortex that deals with physical sensations. The good thing about this is that in order to have a better orgasm, you have to have your partner focus on the penis while you are focused on the sensation that you are getting from their touch.

## Keep Your Feet Warm

This may sound crazy, but scientists have found that men who have cold feet will have a harder time reaching orgasm than those who are wearing socks or have warm feet. When the man is comfortable, he is going to be more relaxed. This relaxation is the key to have better orgasms. If you are afraid of being made fun of for wearing your socks, you can turn the heat up or place them into some warm water before she shows up.

## Sex Positions to Sustain an Erection

Maybe you struggle with maintaining an erection, and that is what keeps you from enjoying your orgasm. There are some positions that can help with this.

One way to help things along is by having your partner straddle you. They will sit on your lap, facing you, and will lean back a bit and slide their pelvis up and down along the penis. You will also tease them with your fingers by rubbing their clit. Once you get hard, you can turn this into seated cowgirl, or you can simply stroke yourself while they continue to rub themselves up and down you.

You can also try the wake-up curl. Morning wood is something that shouldn't be taken for granted. This is the time when testosterone is the highest, so have morning sex. Both of you will be on your side, and you will slide up behind her. This means you won't have to worry about morning breath, and she will have a tighter feeling, which will help keep you hard.

Lastly, you can try the pointer dog. This is like doggy-style, but the woman will spread their legs further apart. This will allow you to pull out whenever you need to slow things down or to stroke yourself to keep the erection going. As you do this, you can continue thrusting your fingers into her.

# Chapter 16: Pregnancy Sex Positions

Some couples think that they can't have sex once pregnant, especially later on in the pregnancy. The truth is, sex at any point during pregnancy can happen as long as everybody remains comfortable. There is no need to worry about your baby hearing things because they don't understand language, and the sounds are very well muffled.

If both parties are okay with it, then you can try some of the following sex positions. All of these positions help keep him off of the belly and will make things easier for the mom-to-be. That said, there are some women who don't feel like having sex. It is up to the hormones, so you will need to go with the flower.

Some of the best positions for you to try during pregnancy are those that will keep the pressure off of the belly and the woman off her back. When on her back, it can cause blood flow compression, which can cause her to end up becoming lightheaded, and can cause other problems. So the next time you want to have sex while pregnant, try these positions:

- Anal Sex

If this is something that the two of you have already been doing, you can continue to do so. Trying anal for the first time while pregnant would not be a good idea since most women experience heightened sensations, so it might not be enjoyable. For those who are used to it, you can try anal in any position that we are going to discuss.

- Seated

This is a lot like the lap dance kama sutra position, except you won't be facing him. He sits in the chair, or wherever, and you will sit on him. This puts her in control of everything.

- Standing

There are two options with this. You can face each other, or he can be behind her. Which one works best is going to depend on how far along she is. Facing each other isn't going to work late in the pregnancy. After the third trimester, he will probably need to be behind. This will limit his thrusting ability, so it helps for those who are experiencing with heightened sensitivity.

- Doggy Style

This will keep her off her back and doesn't add any pressure to the belly as long as she stays propped up. This places the man in control of the movements, so he needs to check in with her to make sure he isn't too rough.

- Spooning

Both of you will be laying on your said facing the same direction. The man has a little more control in this position, but the depth and speed won't be as much as with doggy style.

- Cowgirl or Reverse Cowgirl

This places the women in charge of the movement and will keep pressure off of her belly. This works well for women experiencing extra sensitivity.

You should also have pillows at the ready to help her get comfortable, and pregnancy pillows are great. You may also want to think about using toys and lube.

While you can do most sex positions while pregnant, there are things that you should never do.

- Missionary is not good with the woman on the bottom because it can compress blood flow, especially after the 20-week mark.

- Any prone position where the woman will have to lay on her stomach.

- And you should never blow air up the woman's vagina. This is something you should never do at any time, whether she is pregnant or not.

Having sex during pregnancy can require the two of you to get creative and figure out what is going to work for both of you. What may be comfortable at one time may not be later on. And you never know how the hormones will affect her.

# Chapter 17: Oral Sex Positions

Oral sex can be a great way to get things ready for penetration, or it can be the main event of the night. If you are a woman who is not able to reach an orgasm through penetration alone, oral sex is what you are going to need to get things going. The following positions can give you new ways to perform oral sex so that it doesn't seem like the same old boring oral sex.

## Spiderman

Most blow jobs won't allow you to have a good view, but this position will provide your partner with a full view of your body. You lay down on your back on a bed or table. Your head should dangle over the edge. They will come up behind you and lean over so that you are able to swallow their penis. You will be able to use your hands and mouth. They also have the ability to pinch and rub your nipples or clitoris while you are working on their penis.

## Sidecar

Both of you will lay down your sides facing one another. Then you slide down until his penis is in your face. This could be called a lazy blow job if you want. Blow jobs don't have to kill your knees.

## Leg Up

There are some women who have one side of their vulva that is more sensitive than the other. You will lift up that leg on the side that is more sensitive so that it is exposed. Then you will lick figure eights up and down the vulva to please them.

## Deep V

You will start by laying down on your back at the edge of the bed. Grab your thighs and lift your legs up into a V shape. If you aren't this flexible, then you keep your knees bent and let your legs rest on your chest. He will kneel in front of you and start working on you. They can massage your thighs to help bring more blood into your vulva. This can help you to have an amazing orgasm.

## Cliff Hanger

You sit on the edge of the bed and keep your legs dangling off the edge. He will kneel between your legs and go to work. They will use their hands to play with whatever they want to help heighten your pleasure.

## Sofa So Good

You will start by laying upside down on your couch. Your head and back will be flat on the seat while your legs go over the back. Your partner is going to kneel over your face and facing the back of the couch. You can suck his penis while he licks you.

## Doggy Does Oral

This is a very hot position that you will get to control the pressure and angle of. She will be on her hands and knees, just like in doggy, but he will kneel behind you and perform for her. This is also great for a rim job if you want.

## Hail the Queen

The point of sitting on a person's face is not to actually sit on their face. You simply straddle their head and work your thighs. You hold yourself a few inches over their face while they work on you. They can still reach up and play with breasts, or anything else that they want to.

## Corkscrew

The man will stand for this one as you kneel in front of him. Hold the base of his penis in both hands. Place the penis in your mouth and then tilt your head from side to side as your work up and down.

## Fake Deep Throat

You can get the feel of a deep throat without having to gag by putting some lube on your hand and using it on the part of him that won't fit in your mouth. Move your hand as you would move your mouth. To make this more intense, look deep into their eyes.

## Peace Out

You are going to be sitting in a chair while your partner kneels between your legs. The will place two fingers on each side of the clitoris and make the same motions you would if you were using scissors as they suck and lick the tip of the click. This will isolate the clit from the rest of the genitals and pinpoints the pleasure.

## Swiper

Ask your partner to form some suction on the clit by placing their mouth over the labia and clitoris. Now have them shake their head in circles, side to side, and change the pace up. This is going to mimic how many of us masturbate. You can place some pillows under you to give them better access.

## Supersize Me

Once you have your man right at the brink of an orgasm, stop and gently pull a bit on their testicles to stop them from having an orgasm. Give them a bit to recuperate and then go back to it. Once you have them begging, push a finger or vibrator against their penis and watch what happens.

## Constellation

If oral sex is uncomfortable for you, you can try it on your side. This is great for people who have spasticity in their hips that makes it harder for them to spread the legs during oral sex. This will provide your partner with access to your genitals without having to be a position that causes pain.

## Saddle Straddle

If your partner is more dominant, they will love straddling you as you suck and stroke their penis. You can use your hands and twist up and down their penis, and you lick the tip.

## Live Show

If the two of you are into bondage, you can take charge by sitting them down in a chair and then blindfolding them. You can also take a bit further by tying their arms behind the chair. A safeword should be used. Then you will perform oral sex on them and take them to the edge by not allowing them to have an orgasm until you want them to.

## Deep-Sea Diver

This is a great position for a rim job. This can be introduced in the shower. The receiver stays standing as the giver squats behind them and performing oral sex.

## Butterball

This is another great position for rim jobs. The person receiving needs to be showered and fresh. They will lay down and pull their knees into their chest. This will give the doer the chance to reach the clitoris and breasts of the receive. If the man is the receiver, the woman can play with whatever she wants.

## Shark Fin

Since oral sex doesn't work well underwater, the women will lay down with her hips at the edge of the tub. She will open up her legs but keep her feet in the water and enjoy everything her partner does to her.

# Chapter 18: How to Have Better Sex

While you may not want to think about exercising when you want to have better sex, exercising has the ability to improve your sex life. Athletes train for years for their athletic endeavors, and sex is no exception. Practicing the following exercises can help to improve your strength and flexibility, which could be the answer that you and your partner have been searching for in order to make your sex life better. All of the exercises are things that can help both men and women.

- High Plank to Forearm Plank

Start by getting into a high plank position with your hands under shoulders. You want your body to create a straight line. From here, engage your core and carefully move your right hand and lower down onto your right forearm. Do the same on the left forearm. With control, move your right arm to bring you back up onto your hand, and repeat on the left side.

This helps to build upper body strength.

- Scissor Kicks

Start by laying flat on your back. Move your hands under your hips. Raise both legs straight in the air with your toes pointed. Try to keep your legs as straight as you can, and then engage your core and slowly lower your right leg to the ground. Don't touch the floor. Bring your leg back up and repeat with the other side. This is one rep.

This helps build up strength in the low back and abs and improves flexibility.

- Hydrants

Start on your hands and knees, keeping your wrists under your shoulders and knees under hips. Engage the butt and core and raise your right knee to bring it straight to the side. With control, bring the leg back down. You will do ten reps on one side and then do the other.

This helps to open up your hips and improves upper body strength.

- Wide Squat

Bring your legs into a wide stance and point your toes out. Keep your shoulders over your hips. As you squat down, make sure that your knees stay behind your toes. Press back up through your heels. This is one rep.

This helps build thigh strength and improves flexibility.

- The Bird

Begin by squatting down with your legs together, arms bent, hands together, and chest high. Keeping this low position, open up your left knee to the side and take a short step to the left. While you step, rotate your chest open to the left and open your arms so that the left arm goes behind you, and the right arm stays straight out in front.

Bring your left foot back to the starting position and bring both arms forward. Do this on the right side and return to the starting position. This is a single rep.

This will help tone up the upper back, calves, glutes, and quads, as well as improving flexibility. This is particularly helpful for women because it can help with woman-on-top positions.

- Squat with Knee Dip

Begin in a play squat position with your legs wider than shoulder-width and your toes turned out. Bring your arms out in from of you and then squat down. As you push back up, you will have all of your weight on your right foot. Allow your left leg to swivel on the ball of your foot so that the knee turns into the center. Bring the left arm back as you do this.

Turn the leg back out and squat back down. Repeat this movement on the right side. This should be one long fluid motion. One on each side counts as a single rep.

This helps to loosen up the hips, strengthen the obliques, abs, and legs, and helps your rhythm.

- Drop It Low

Begin by standing straight with your heels together, and toes pointed out. Clasp your hands together in front of you with your palms facing down. Making sure your shoulders stay over your hips, allow your heels to come, and your knees to point out to the sides slightly as you start to squat down.

As you move down, raise your hands over your head. Engage the core and then push yourself back up through your feet as you bring your hands back down to come to the starting position.

This will help to open up your hips, strengthen the core, butt, and thighs, and improve balance.

- Hip Swivel

To perform this exercise, begin by standing with your legs should width apart and keep your knees soft. Keep your elbows close to your side, bend your arms, and take your arms out to the side.

Rotate your hips to the right and come up on your toes on your right foot, and allow your butt to pop out to the left. From here, drop your right heel and swivel your hips to the left, bringing your left foot up on your toes. You will be drawing a half-circle behind you with your butt and engaging your core. One-half circle to each side is one rep.

This move helps to loosen up your butt and hips and tightens up the core. It also helps to improve your rhythm if you do this to the beat of some music.

Now that you have these exercises, you can turn on your favorite workout playlist and perform three sets of ten reps for each of these exercises.

# Conclusion

Thank you for making it through to the end of the book, let's hope it was informative and able to provide you with all of the tools you need to achieve your goals whatever they may be.

The next step is to start trying some of these new positions and games to improve your sex life. One of the easiest places for most couples to start is with the massages. It is a very easy way to bring both of you together and to help get you both into the mood. You could even head out and purchase some massage oils to improve the experience. You can then start to work your way into trying some of the foreplay games and sex positions. If dirty talk is something that you have never done, that could be something that the two of you may want to try out. The possibilities are endless as to what you both can do. The main thing is to make sure that both of you are in agreement with what you want to try.

Finally, if you found this book useful in any way, a review on Amazon is always appreciated!

# Description

Do you want to spice up your sex life and improve your relationship? Are you tired of the same old positions night after night? Have you always been a little intrigued by the idea of kama sutra? If you answered yes to any of these questions, then you are going to want to continue reading.

Sex has always been a hush-hush subject because of outdated beliefs and such. This has led to couples getting stuck in a rut when it comes to their sex life. They don't feel that it is "right" to talk to people about their sex life. Times are changing, and more and more people are comfortable talking about their sex life, and that is a good thing. This makes sex less taboo and enables couples to expand their sex repertoire. This new awakening doesn't necessarily mean that couples will find the answer they want or need from people they talk to, though, and that's what this book is here to do.

This book has been brought together to provide information about sex to help couples who are tired of the same old thing every night. Foreplay, that's is the one word most couples dread. For some reason, this is the area where couples end up failing, yet we all know that it is extremely important, especially for women. It helps to place people in the right state of mind and gets things warmed up, so to speak. This isn't the only problem some couples have in their sex life. Sometimes it's simply that things have turned monotonous. This is understandable, especially when you and your partner have been together for a while. It is very easy to stick with the same things because you know what one another likes, or because it is easy. But you both likely feel bored and can easily pass on sex due to the boredom. But things don't have to stay that way, though. You can easily bring the spark back into your life, whether through foreplay or new positions.

This book is here to teach you how you can improve your sex life. In this book, you will learn:

- Why you should bring kama sutra and tantra into your bedroom

- The best sex positions for men and women

- The best sex positions to bring the two of you together

- Sex tips for the beginner

- Foreplay games to get things heated up

- How to practice couples massages

- The best way to start using dirty talk without feeling weird

... And much more.

I get that you might still be skeptical that this book can help improve your sex life. Even if you have tried new things to try and spice up your sex life without success, this book can teach you things that you may not have thought about. The information in this book can be applied to anybody's sex life. You'll even find that within the descriptions of various sex positions, there will be warnings, so you are guided throughout the entire process. I'm certain that if you buy this book today, you won't regret it.

Now is the time to make the decision. If you are serious about changing your sex life, scroll up now, and click "buy now."

www.ingramcontent.com/pod-product-compliance
Lightning Source LLC
Chambersburg PA
CBHW050728030426
42336CB00012B/1461